Personal Information

Name: _____

Department: _____

Home Address: _____

_____

Phone Number: _____

Pager Number: _____ Fax Number: _____

Cell Phone Number: _____

E-mail Address: _____

Personal Health Data

Date of Last Tetanus Booster:

Hepatitis B Vaccination Dates

   First: _____

   Second: _____

   Third: _____

W0113636

Date of Last Hepatitis B Booster: _____

Date of Last Titer Test and Results: _____

Date of Last TB Test: _____

Physician's Phone Number: _____

Dentist's Phone Number: _____

Certifications

EMT Certification Number: _____ Expiration Date: _____

National Reg. EMT Certification Number: _____ Expiration Date: _____

CPR Expiration Date: _____

Date of Last EMT Refresher: _____

Firefighter Certification Number: _____ Expiration Date: _____

Hazardous Materials Level: _____ Expiration Date: _____

Date of Last Hazardous Materials Refresher: _____

1   Personal Data

Specialty Certifications/Training Courses

Course Name:_____ Date:_____

_____
_____
_____
_____
_____
_____
_____
_____
_____
_____
_____
_____
_____
_____
_____
_____
_____
_____
_____
_____
_____
_____
_____
_____
_____
_____
_____

Scene Size-up

Scene Safety

Take standard precautions.

Determine:

- If the scene is safe
- Mechanism of injury (MOI)/nature of illness (NOI)
- Number of patients
- If additional/specialized resources are necessary

Primary Assessment

Identify and treat immediate or potential life threats.

- Form a general impression of the patient.
- Assess the level of consciousness.
- Assess airway and breathing.
  - Identify and treat life threats.
  - Obtain a patent airway.
  - Provide supplemental oxygen.
  - Ventilate if appropriate.
- Assess circulation.
  - Identify and treat life threats.
  - Assess the patient's pulse.
  - Assess the patient's skin color, temperature, and condition.
  - Assess and control external bleeding.
- Perform a rapid scan.
- Determine the priority of patient care.
  - **Identify high-priority patients (see the next section).**
- Make a transport decision.
- Consider advanced life support (ALS) intervention.

High-Priority Patients

- Difficulty breathing
- Poor general impression
- Unresponsive with no gag or cough reflexes

- Severe chest pain
- Pale skin or other signs of poor perfusion
- Complicated childbirth
- Uncontrolled bleeding
- Responsive but unable to follow commands
- Severe pain in any area of the body
- Inability to move any part of the body

History Taking

- Investigate the chief complaint (history of present illness).
- Obtain the SAMPLE history.

Secondary Assessment

- If unable to perform a secondary assessment at the scene, perform it in the ambulance en route to the hospital. In some situations, the EMT may not be able to perform a secondary assessment because of life threats.

Assess Vital Signs
Full-Body Scan

- Perform a full-body scan on patients who have a significant MOI, who are unconscious, or who are in critical condition.
- This systematic head-to-toe examination identifies hidden injuries or causes that may not have been found during the rapid scan.

Focused Assessment

- Perform a focused assessment on patients who have a nonsignificant MOI or who are responsive.
- Base the area of assessment on the chief complaint.

Reassessment

- Repeat the primary assessment.
- Reassess vital signs.
- Reassess the chief complaint.
- Recheck interventions.
- Identify and treat changes in the patient's condition.

- Reassessment time intervals:
  - Stable patients: repeat and record findings every 15 minutes
  - Unstable patients: repeat and record findings every 5 minutes

Table 1 Normal Pulse Rates

Age	Range (beats/min)
Infant: 1 month to 1 year	100 to 160
Toddler: 1 to 3 years	90 to 150
Preschool age: 3 to 6 years	80 to 140
School age: 6 to 12 years	70 to 120
Adolescent: 12 to 18 years	60 to 100
Adult	60 to 100

Table 2 Normal Respiration Rate Ranges

Adults and adolescents	12 to 20
Children	15 to 30
Infants	25 to 50

Note: Ranges presented in other courses may vary.

Table 3 Normal Range for Blood Pressure

Age	Range (mm Hg)
Adults	90 to 140 (systolic)
Children (ages 1 to 8 years)	80 to 110 (systolic)
Infants (newborn to age 1 year)	50 to 95 (systolic)

Patient Assessment Acronyms

AVPU
A = Alert
V = Responds to verbal stimuli
P = Responds to painful stimuli
U = Unresponsive

SAMPLE History
Obtain information from the patient or, if the patient is unresponsive, from family, friends, or bystanders.

Signs and symptoms (also look for medical ID tag):
- **Sign: something the EMT sees, hears, or feels (example: skin color, wheezing, swelling)**
- **Symptom: something the patient tells the EMT (example: pain, shortness of breath)**

Allergies (to medications, foods, environment)

Medications (currently or recently taking, including over-the-counter remedies)

Pertinent past medical history

Last oral intake (solid or liquid)

Events leading up to injury or illness

OPQRST
Onset

Provocation (What makes it better or worse?)

Quality

Radiation

Severity

Time (duration)

DCAP-BTLS

Deformities

Contusions

Abrasions

Punctures/penetrations

Burns

Tenderness

Lacerations

Swelling

Coma Scales

Table 4 Adult Glasgow Coma Scale (GCS)

Physical Sign	Response	Points	Score
Eye opening	Spontaneous In response to speech In response to pain None	4 3 2 1	
Best motor response	Obeys command Localizes pain Withdraws to pain Abnormal flexion Abnormal extension None	6 5 4 3 2 1	
Best verbal response	Oriented conversation Confused conversation Inappropriate words Incomprehensible sounds None	5 4 3 2 1	
Total	Apply this score to GCS portion of trauma score	3-15	
Score: Possible 3-15, decreasing with injury severity			

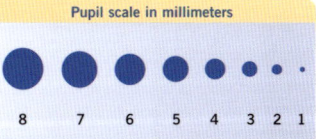

Pupil scale in millimeters

8 7 6 5 4 3 2 1

Signs and Symptoms

Closed Abdominal Injuries

- Kehr sign (pain in the left shoulder)
- Tearing pain
- Acute abdominal pain
- Rebound tenderness
- Guarding
- Abdominal distention
- Bruising and discoloration
- Abrasions
- Presence of deformity on palpation

Open Abdominal Injuries

- Abdominal pain
- Obvious open wounds
- Tachycardia
- Signs of shock
- Changes in mental status
- Abdominal distention

Management

Closed Abdominal Injuries

- Place the patient in a position of comfort.
- Administer high-flow oxygen to the patient.
- Treat the patient for shock.
- Transport the patient to a trauma center that has a surgeon.

Open Abdominal Injuries

- Inspect the patient's back and sides for exit wounds.
- Apply a dry, sterile dressing to open wounds.
- Stabilize any penetrating objects in place.
- If the patient has an evisceration, apply a moist, sterile dressing over the wound and cover the moist, sterile dressing with a bandage.
- Monitor the patient for signs of shock.

- If the patient shows signs of shock, administer high-flow supplemental oxygen and treat for shock.
- Keep the patient warm with blankets.
- Provide prompt transport.

Abdominal Pain

Signs and Symptoms

- Nausea and vomiting
- Diarrhea
- Fever
- Weakness
- Dizziness
- Painful or frequent urination
- Referred pain, such as pain in the left shoulder (Kehr's sign), or Murphy's sign (severe upper right quadrant pain)

Management

- Administer oxygen.
- Treat the patient for shock.
- Place the patient in a position of comfort.
- Give the patient nothing by mouth.
- Reassess the patient's condition for signs of deterioration.
- Transport the patient to a hospital.

Altered Mental Status

Signs and Symptoms

- The patient's level of consciousness can range from alert but confused to unconscious.
- Compare the patient's level of consciousness to the patient's baseline.
- The causes of altered mental status include:
  - Hypoglycemia
  - Head injury (page 24)
  - Poisoning (page 28)

Management

- Determine the cause of the patient's altered mental status.
- Maintain the patient's airway and administer oxygen.
- If there are signs of trauma, immobilize the patient's spine.
- Transport the patient to the appropriate facility.

Amputation

Signs and Symptoms

An extremity is completely or partially severed from the body.

Management

Partial Amputation

- Immobilize the part with bulky compression dressings and a splint to prevent further injury.
- Control any bleeding from the stump.
- Apply a tourniquet if bleeding cannot be controlled.
- Transport the patient to the appropriate hospital.

Complete Amputation

- Wrap the clean part in a sterile dressing and place it in a plastic bag.
- Follow local protocols on preserving amputated parts.
- Put the bag on a bed of ice in a cool container.
- Control bleeding and apply an appropriate bandage.
- Transport the amputated part with the patient to the appropriate hospital.

Anaphylaxis

Signs and Symptoms

- Hives
- Stridor
- Bronchospasm
- Shock
- Oral or facial edema

Management

- Remove the offending agent.
- Maintain the patient's airway, administer oxygen, and assist with ventilation as needed.
- Administer an epinephrine auto-injector, per local protocol.
- Rapidly transport the patient.

 Asthma

Signs and Symptoms

- Wheezing on inspiration/expiration
- Bronchospasm
- Increased respiration rate

Management

- Suction any mucus from the patient's airway and administer oxygen. Do not withhold oxygen for longer than:
  - Adults—15 seconds
  - Children—10 seconds
  - Infants—5 seconds
- Assist the patient to use his or her prescribed inhaler, per local protocol.
- Assist the patient's ventilations if needed, providing about 10–12 shallow breaths/min.
- Patients with a prolonged asthma attack require oxygen and immediate transport.
- ALS management should be considered per local protocols.

Burns

Signs and Symptoms

Burn Classifications

- **Superficial burns** involve only the epidermis.
  - Reddened skin
  - Pain at the site

- **Partial-thickness burns** involve the epidermis and the dermis, but not the underlying tissue.
  - White to red moist and mottled skin
  - Blisters
  - Intense pain
- **Full-thickness burns** extend through all the dermal layers and may also involve subcutaneous layers, muscle, bone, or organs.
  - The skin may appear white, dark brown, or charred.
  - The skin is dry and leathery and hard to the touch.
  - The patient reports little or no pain, except at the periphery of the burn.

Severity Chart

- **Minor burns**
  - Full-thickness burns involving less than 2% of total body surface
  - Partial-thickness burns involving less than 15% of total body surface
  - Superficial burns involving less than 50% of total body surface
- **Moderate burns**
  - Full-thickness burns involving 2% to 10% of total body surface, excluding hands, feet, face, genitalia, or upper airway
  - Partial-thickness burns involving 15% to 30% of total body surface
  - Superficial burns involving more than 50% of total body surface
- **Critical burns**
  - Full-thickness burns involving hands, feet, face, genitalia, upper airway, or circumferential burns of other areas
  - Burns associated with respiratory injury
  - Full-thickness burns involving more than 10% of total body surface

- Partial-thickness burns involving more than 30% of total body surface
- Patients younger than 5 years or older than 55 years who meet moderate burn criteria for young adults
- Burns complicated by a fracture

Signs and Symptoms of Respiratory Burns

- Cough
- Singed nasal hairs
- Difficulty breathing
- Hoarseness
- Sooty sputum
- Facial burns
- Soot around mouth and nose

Management

- Stop the burning process. Remove any smoldering clothing and jewelry.
- Cool the burn area with cool, sterile water when appropriate.
- Administer high-flow oxygen to the patient, and continually reassess the airway for problems, especially if there are signs of respiratory burns.
- Rapidly estimate the burn's severity using the Rule of Nines (page 15).
- Cover the burn area with a dry, sterile dressing to prevent contamination.
  - Do not break blisters.
  - Do not place ointments or lotions on the burn.
- Treat the patient for shock.
- Prevent heat loss in the patient with blankets.
- Provide prompt transport per local protocol.

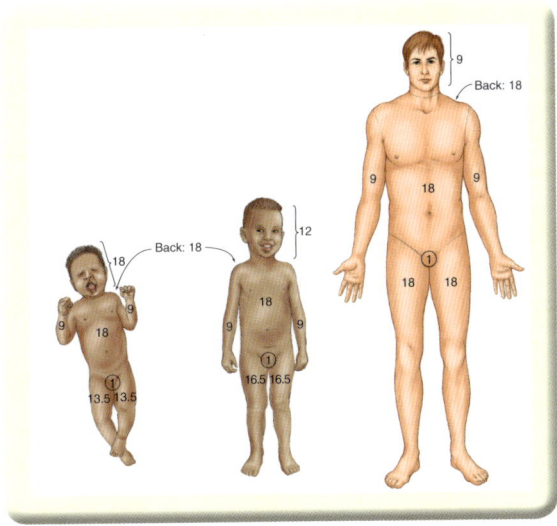

The size of the patient's palm equals approximately 1% of his or her body surface.

Cardiac Arrest

Signs and Symptoms
Absent or barely palpable pulse

Management

- **Do not use an automated external defibrillator (AED) on patients younger than 1 month of age.** Whenever possible, use an AED with pediatric-sized pads and a dose-attenuating system (energy reducer) on patients between 1 month and 8 years of age.
- Take standard precautions.
- Quickly question rescuers or bystanders about arrest events.
- Direct rescuers to stop cardiopulmonary resuscitation (CPR).
- Verify the absence of a pulse.
- If there is no pulse, perform five cycles (about 2 minutes) of CPR (pages 40–41). If two EMTs are present, one continues CPR while the other sets up the AED.
- Turn on the defibrillator power.
- Connect the defibrillator to the patient. Place one pad on the upper right chest and the other over the lower part of the left side of the chest.
- **Discontinue CPR and ensure everyone is standing clear of the patient.**
- Initiate analysis of rhythm.
- **If appropriate, deliver a shock.**
- After the shock is delivered, immediately resume CPR, beginning with chest compressions.
- After five cycles (about 2 minutes) of CPR, reanalyze the cardiac rhythm.
  - If appropriate, deliver another shock and immediately resume CPR.
  - If no shock is advised, immediately resume CPR.

- After 2 minutes of CPR, reanalyze the cardiac rhythm, then repeat the cycle of 2 minutes of CPR, one shock (if indicated), and 2 minutes of CPR.
- Transport the patient and contact medical control as needed.

Critical Points
- Immediately evaluate the need for use of an AED.
- Be familiar with proper operation of the AED being used.
- Ensure initiation and resumption of ventilations and compressions at appropriate times.
- Ensure that all individuals are clear of the patient before delivering shocks.
- If a patient who must be defibrillated is wearing a nitroglycerin patch on his or her chest, remove the nitroglycerin patch before defibrillating.
- If defibrillation needs to be performed in the back of an ambulance, stop the ambulance before analyzing the cardiac rhythm and delivering a shock.
- If the patient regains a pulse following defibrillation, keep the AED attached to the patient during transport in case the patient arrests again. (**Note:** The defibrillator may be turned off to avoid accidental delivery of a shock.)

Chest Injuries

Signs and Symptoms
- Pain at the injury site
- Pain that increases with breathing
- Bruising to the chest wall
- Crepitus with palpation to the chest
- Any penetrating injury to the chest
- Dyspnea
- Hemoptysis (coughing up blood)
- Unequal chest rise
- Rapid, weak pulse

- Low blood pressure
- Cyanosis around the lips or fingertips

Management

- If there are signs of trauma, immobilize the patient's spine.
- Maintain an open airway and be prepared to suction the patient.
- Insert an airway adjunct and assist with ventilations if necessary.
- Administer high-flow oxygen if internal bleeding is suspected.
- Control any bleeding.
- Apply an occlusive dressing over any penetrating trauma to the chest wall.
- Apply a bulky dressing to stabilize any flail segments.
- Be prepared to provide positive-pressure ventilation.
- Treat the patient for any signs of shock.
- Do not delay transport of a seriously injured trauma patient to complete nonlifesaving treatments; complete those types of treatment en route.

Chest Pain

Signs and Symptoms

- Sudden onset of:
  - Weakness
  - Nausea
  - Sweating
- Squeezing or crushing chest pain
- Pain or pressure in the:
  - Lower jaw
  - Arms
  - Abdomen
  - Neck
- Irregular heartbeat
- Syncope
- Dyspnea
- Pink, frothy sputum

Management

- Have the patient sit or put him or her in a seated position.
- Loosen all tight clothing.
- Administer oxygen.
- Administer low-dose aspirin and assist with nitroglycerin, per local protocol.
- Promptly transport the patient.

Childbirth

Begin transport unless delivery is anticipated within minutes. Position the patient on her left side if she is in her last trimester.

Signs and Symptoms

- Consider delivery imminent if:
  - Contractions are less than 3 minutes apart and longer than 45 seconds in duration.
  - The mother feels the need to push.
  - The infant is crowning.
- If this is the patient's first delivery, the time for actual delivery may take longer than subsequent deliveries would.

Management

Normal Delivery

- Support the baby's head and use gentle pressure to prevent an explosive birth.
- If the amniotic sac has not broken, puncture it and push it away from the newborn's head and mouth.
- As the baby's head is delivered, check for the umbilical cord around the baby's neck. If it is around the neck, loosen it and slip it over the baby's head or clamp and cut it.
- Suction the newborn's mouth and nose with a bulb syringe.
- Compress the bulb before placing it in the baby's mouth.
- Suction the mouth/oropharynx first, then each nostril.
- To deliver the shoulders, guide the head downward, then upward.

- Dry the infant and wrap the baby in a warm blanket with the head slightly lower than the trunk.
- Keep the baby warm (pay special attention to the baby's head).
- Keep the infant at the same level as the mother's vagina until the cord is cut.
- Place cord clamps after pulsations in the umbilical cord cease. Place the first clamp approximately four fingerbreadths from the baby and the second several inches farther away from the first clamp.
- Record the Apgar score findings 1 minute and 5 minutes after birth.

Table 5 Apgar Scores

Sign	0	1	2
Appearance (skin color)	Completely blue or pale	Body pink; hands and feet blue	Completely pink
Pulse rate (heart rate)	Absent	< 100 beats/min	> 100 beats/min
Grimace (irritability)	No response	Weak cry in response to stimulus	Cries and tries to move foot away from finger snapped against its sole
Activity (muscle tone)	Completely limp	Makes weak attempts to resist straightening	Resists attempts to straighten hips and knees
Respirations (respiratory effort)	Absent	Slow	Rapid
7-10: Excellent condition; supportive care only **4-6:** Moderately depressed **0-3:** Severely depressed; immediate resuscitation needed			

Deliver the Placenta

- Delivery of the placenta should occur within a few minutes after childbirth but may take as long as 30 minutes.
- Blood loss of less than 500 mL is usual.
- Once the placenta delivers, the bleeding should stop.
- Allowing the baby to nurse or massaging the mother's lower abdomen may speed delivery of the placenta.
- Never pull on the end of the umbilical cord.
- Administer oxygen and provide prompt transport if:
  - The placenta has not delivered after 30 minutes.
  - More than 500 mL of bleeding occurs before delivery of the placenta.
  - Significant bleeding occurs after delivery of the placenta.

Breech Presentation

- Place the mother on high-flow oxygen.
- Provide emergency care and call for ALS assistance.
- Never attempt to assist delivery by pulling on the newborn.
- If the body delivers, support the infant to help prevent explosive delivery of the head.
- As the head is delivering, place gloved fingers into the mother's vagina to form a "V" to keep the walls of the vagina from compressing the newborn's airway.
- If the mother does not deliver within 10 minutes of buttocks presentation, provide prompt transport.

Prolapsed Umbilical Cord

- Place the mother on high-flow oxygen.
- Elevate the mother's hips. Consider placing the mother in the knee–chest or Trendelenburg's position.
- Insert a sterile gloved hand into the mother's vagina to gently push the newborn's head away from the umbilical cord.
- Do not attempt to push the umbilical cord back into the mother's vagina.
- Cover any portion of the exposed cord with moist, sterile dressings.
- Transport rapidly.

Limb Presentation

- Place the mother on high-flow oxygen.
- Place the mother on her back and elevate her pelvis.
- Do not pull on the limb.
- Do not attempt to push the limb back into the mother's vagina.

Croup

Signs and Symptoms

- Dyspnea (shortness of breath)
- Chest tightness
- Stridor (high-pitched sound on inspiration)
- Seal-bark cough
- Low-grade fever

Management

- Administer humidified oxygen to the patient if it is available.
- Transport the patient promptly to the hospital.

Drowning

Management

- Use the "reach, throw, and row, and only then go" guideline to safely remove the patient from the water.
- Ensure a patent and clear airway.
- Begin CPR if pulse and breathing are absent (pages 40, 41).
- If pulse and breathing are present, administer oxygen and assist ventilations if needed.
- Keep the patient warm and transport.

Epiglottitis

Signs and Symptoms

- Very sore throat
- High fever

- Tripod position
- Drooling
- Stridor (high-pitched sound on inspiration)

Management

- Keep the patient in a position of comfort.
- Administer high-flow oxygen.
- *Do not* put anything into the patient's mouth, including implements such as airway adjuncts and suctioning tubes; doing so can create a complete airway obstruction.
- Transport the patient promptly.

Head Injuries

Signs and Symptoms

- Lacerations, contusions, or hematomas to the scalp
- Soft area or depression on palpation
- Visible fractures or deformities of the skull
- Bruising around the eyes or behind the ears
- Clear or pink cerebrospinal fluid leakage from a scalp wound, the nose, or the ear
- Loss of sensation or motor function
- A period of unconsciousness
- Amnesia
- Seizures
- Numbness or tingling in the extremities
- Irregular respirations
- Dizziness
- Visual complaints
- Abnormal behavior
- Nausea or vomiting

Management

- Establish and maintain a patent airway.
- Administer high-flow oxygen and support ventilations, if needed.

- Consider the need for spinal immobilization.
- Control bleeding.
- Begin CPR if necessary (pages 40, 41).
- Assess the patient's baseline level of consciousness and monitor it.
- Assess and treat any other injuries.
- Anticipate and manage vomiting.
- Be prepared for convulsions and changes in the patient's condition.
- Transport the patient promptly and with extreme care.

Hyperthermia

Signs and Symptoms
Heat Cramps
Cramping in the leg or abdomen
Heat Exhaustion
- Dizziness, weakness, faintness
- Change in the level of consciousness
- Muscle cramping
- Cold, clammy skin with ashen pallor
- Rapid and weak pulse
- Normal or slightly elevated body temperature
Heatstroke
- Hot, dry, flushed skin
- Body temperature of 106°F (41°C) or more
- Decreasing level of consciousness

Management
- Remove the patient from the hot environment.
- Loosen any tight clothing.
Heat Cramps
- Administer high-flow oxygen.
- Rest the cramping muscles by having the patient sit or lie down.
- Replace fluids by mouth.
- Cool the patient with cool water spray or fan the patient.

Heat Exhaustion
- Administer oxygen.
- Place the patient in a supine position and fan him or her.
- If the patient is fully alert, give water by mouth.
- If nausea develops, transport the patient on his or her side.

Heatstroke
- Set air conditioning to the maximum cooling setting.
- Remove the patient's clothing.
- Administer high-flow oxygen and assist with ventilations if needed.
- Apply cool packs to the patient's neck, groin, and armpits.
- Cover the patient with wet towels or sheets or spray the patient with cool water and fan him or her.
- Aggressively and repeatedly fan the patient.
- Provide immediate transport and notify the hospital.

 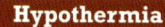

Hypothermia

Signs and Symptoms

Core Temperature 93° to 95°F (34° to 35°C)
- Alert
- Shivering
- Foot stamping
- Rapid pulse and respirations
- Blue lips or fingertips

Core Temperature 89° to 92°F (32° to 33°C)
- Shivering stops
- Loss of coordination
- Muscle stiffness

Core Temperature 80° to 88°F (27° to 31°C)
- Decreased level of consciousness
- Poor coordination
- Memory loss
- Reduced sensation to touch

- Rigid muscles
- Weak pulse and very slow respirations

Core Temperature < 80°F (< 27°C)
- Cardiorespiratory activity may cease.
- The patient's pupils may be slow to react.
- The patient may appear to be dead.

Management
- Never assume that a cold, pulseless patient is dead.
- Establish and maintain a patent airway.
- Provide oxygen.
- Monitor for vomiting and protect against aspiration.
- Carefully move the patient to a protected environment.
- Remove any wet clothing.
- Place dry blankets over and under the patient.
- Handle the patient gently. With severe hypothermia, rough handling can cause ventricular fibrillation.
- In the event of mild hypothermia, begin active rewarming.
- In the event of moderate or severe hypothermia, prevent further heat loss and follow local protocols.

◆ Orthopaedic Injuries

Signs and Symptoms
Dislocation
- Marked deformity
- Swelling
- Pain
- Tenderness
- Loss of joint motion
- Numbness or impaired circulation to the limb

Fracture
- Deformity
- Point tenderness
- Guarding

- Swelling
- Bruising
- Crepitus (grating or grinding)
- False motion
- Exposed fragments
- Pain
- Locked joint

Sprain

- Point tenderness
- Swelling and bruising at the point of injury
- Pain that prevents the patient from moving or using the limb
- Joint instability

Strain

- Minor swelling at the injury site
- Increased pain with passive movement

Management

- Consider the need for spinal immobilization.
- Open, clear, and maintain the patient's airway.
- Administer high-flow oxygen and ensure adequate ventilation.
- Control any bleeding.
- Treat the patient for shock.
- Cover open wounds with a dry, sterile dressing and apply pressure to control bleeding.
- Apply a splint and elevate the patient's extremity.
- Apply cold packs if there is swelling. Do not place them directly on the skin.
- Position the patient for transport.
- Transport the patient to the appropriate treatment facility.

Poisoning

Signs and Symptoms

- Burn injuries and/or discoloration at the patient's mouth
- Dilated or constricted pupils

- Depressed respiratory rate
- Cyanosis
- Rapid or weakened pulse
- Seizures
- Altered mental status

Management

- Establish and maintain a patent airway.
- Provide high-flow oxygen.
- Monitor for vomiting and protect against aspiration.
- Request ALS when necessary.
- Take all containers, bottles, and labels of poisons to the hospital.
- If the poisoning is the result of alcohol, opioids, sedative-hypnotics, or abused inhalants, monitor the patient's level of consciousness and airway.
- Patients who have abused inhalants are prone to seizures and ventricular fibrillation.
- If the poisoning was caused by stimulants or anticholinergics, monitor the patient for hypertension (high blood pressure) or other cardiovascular effects.
- For patients with plant poisoning, contact the regional poison center for assistance in identifying the plant.
- For patients with food poisoning, transport the suspected food with the patient.
- Administer activated charcoal according to local protocol.

Psychiatric Emergencies

- If there is any reason to believe that the patient may be violent, do not approach the scene without law enforcement officials.
- Approach the patient with caution and monitor the patient's behavior.
- Be aware of your surroundings and watch for possible weapons.

- If you are accompanied by law enforcement personnel, ask them to check the patient for weapons.
- Speak to the patient in a normal tone of voice and do not raise your voice.

Management

- Manage any life threats to the patient's ABCs.
- Administer high-flow oxygen.
- Without an underlying medical or trauma cause, there is little hands-on care to perform.
- If you have a reasonable belief that the patient may harm himself, herself, or others, contact law enforcement.
- If restraint is required:
  - Consult with medical control.
  - Ensure that law enforcement personnel are at the scene.
  - Make sure there are at least four people present.
  - Only use approved restraint devices.
  - Never restrain a patient in the prone position.
  - Check for circulation in the patient's extremities during transport.

Respiratory Distress, Adult

Signs and Symptoms

- Difficulty breathing
- Shortness of breath
- Shallow breathing
- Chest pain or discomfort
- Accessory muscle retraction
- Patient in the tripod position
- Cough, either productive or nonproductive
- Fever or chills

Asthma (page 12)

Bronchitis

- Chronic cough
- Wheezing
- Cyanosis
- Productive cough

Chronic Obstructive Pulmonary Disease (COPD)

- Shortness of breath
- Wheezing
- Chronic coughing
- Sputum
- Long expirations
- Abnormal breath sounds
- Rales
- Crackles
- Rhonchi
- Wheezes

Epiglottitis (page 23)

Foreign Body Obstruction

- Weak or absent cough
- Decreasing level of consciousness
- Cyanosis

Pneumonia

- Dyspnea
- Chills, fever
- Cough
- Dark sputum

Pneumothorax

- Sudden chest pain with dyspnea
- Decreased lung sounds on the affected side

Management

- Manage life threats to the patient's ABCs and ensure the delivery of high-flow oxygen.
- Patients breathing at a rate of less than 8 breaths/min or greater than 30 breaths/min should have ventilations assisted with a bag-mask device.
- Continually assess the patient's mental status and provide emotional support as needed.
- Transport in the position of comfort.
- For all respiratory emergencies, make sure you have taken the appropriate standard precautions, including the use of a HEPA respirator.

Bronchitis

- Administer oxygen to the patient.
- Monitor the patient's vital signs.
- Transport the patient to the hospital.

Chronic Obstructive Pulmonary Disease (COPD)

- Assist the patient to use his or her prescribed inhaler, if he or she has one.
- Document the time and effect on the patient with each use.
- Transport patients with chronic obstructive pulmonary disease (COPD) as promptly as possible to the emergency department.
- Allow the patient to sit upright if this is comfortable; breathing may be difficult when he or she is lying down.
- Treat the patient with high-flow oxygen via nonrebreathing mask at 15 L/min and watch for the reverse breathing reflex; too much oxygen can eliminate the patient's stimulus to breathe.

Foreign Body Obstruction

Remove the foreign body that is causing the obstruction.

Pneumonia

- Administer oxygen to the patient.
- Monitor the patient's vital signs.
- Transport the patient to the hospital.

Pneumothorax

- Place the patient in a position of comfort.
- Support the patient's ABCs.
- Provide prompt transport.
- Monitor the patient carefully.
- Be prepared to assist ventilations and provide CPR if necessary.

Respiratory Distress, Pediatric

Signs and Symptoms

- Nasal flaring
- Grunting respirations
- Wheezing
- Stridor
- Accessory muscle use
- Retractions
- Tripod position
- Asthma (page 12)
- Croup (page 23)
- Epiglottitis (page 23)

Foreign Body Obstruction

- Weak or absent cough
- Decreasing level of consciousness
- Cyanosis

Management

- Maintain the patient's airway.
- Suction the patient's airway as necessary.
- Administer oxygen to the patient and ventilate as necessary.
- Place the patient in a position of comfort.
- Transport the patient calmly and rapidly.

Foreign Body Obstruction

- Remove the foreign body that is causing the obstruction.

Seizures

Signs and Symptoms

- Cyanosis (bluish lips, tongue, and skin)
- Traumatic injury as a result of a fall
- Incontinence
- Loss of consciousness
- Labored breathing
- Weakness of one side of the body
- Lethargy
- Confusion

Management

- Ensure an open airway, but *do not* place anything into the patient's mouth.
- Administer high-flow oxygen via a nonrebreathing mask.
- Obtain blood glucose level per local protocol.
- Do not restrain a patient having a seizure.
- Provide emotional support.
- Transport the patient to a hospital.

Shock

Signs and Symptoms

Cardiogenic Shock

- Chest pain
- Irregular pulse
- Weak pulse
- Low blood pressure
- Cyanosis (lips, under nails)
- Cool, clammy skin
- Anxiety
- Rales (fluid in the lungs)

Neurogenic Shock
- Bradycardia (slow pulse)
- Low blood pressure
- Suspected neck injury

Hypovolemic Shock
- Rapid, weak pulse
- Low blood pressure
- Change in mental status
- Cyanosis (lips, under nails)
- Cool, clammy skin
- Increased respiratory rate

Septic Shock
- Warm skin
- Tachycardia
- Low blood pressure

Management

Cardiogenic Shock
- Administer high-flow oxygen via a nonrebreathing mask.
- Place the patient in a sitting or semisitting position to assist breathing.
- Do not administer nitroglycerin if blood pressure is low; contact medical control.
- Keep the patient calm, request ALS if available, and transport promptly.
- Keep alert for the need to assist with ventilation, perform CPR, or defibrillate.

Neurogenic Shock
- Maintain cervical spine stabilization and airway control with a modified jaw thrust.
- Provide oxygen and assist breathing as necessary.
- Provide spinal immobilization.
- Prevent body heat loss.
- Transport the patient promptly to a trauma center.

Hypovolemic Shock

- Focus on preventing further blood or fluid loss.
- Manage threats to the ABCs.
- Control external bleeding with direct pressure, pressure dressings, and tourniquets.
- Internal bleeding is difficult to manage. Splinting injured extremities may slow blood loss.
- Place the patient on a long backboard.
- Administer high-flow oxygen.
- Do not delay transport to a trauma center.

Septic Shock

- Assess and manage life threats to the ABCs.
- Administer high-flow oxygen.
- Prevent heat loss.
- Transport the patient as promptly as possible.

Soft-Tissue Injuries: Closed Injuries

Signs and Symptoms

- Bruising
- Swelling
- Pain

Management

- Ensure an open airway and adequate ventilation.
- Monitor and treat for shock.
- Treat a closed, soft-tissue injury by applying RICE, which is an acronym for rest, ice, compression, and elevation.
  - Rest—keep the patient quiet and comfortable.
  - Ice—apply to constrict blood vessels and reduce pain.
  - Compression—compress blood vessels to slow bleeding.
  - Elevation—raise the injured part above the level of the heart to decrease swelling.
- Splint the extremity to decrease bleeding and pain.

Soft-Tissue Injuries: Open Injuries

Signs and Symptoms

- Bleeding
- Exposed tissue
- Swelling
- Deformity

Management

- Ensure an open airway and adequate ventilation.
- Apply an occlusive dressing to open chest injuries.
- Apply a dry, sterile dressing over the wound and apply direct pressure to control bleeding.
- Maintain pressure and secure the dressing with a bandage.
- If bleeding cannot be controlled in an extremity with direct pressure, apply a tourniquet.
- Splint an injured extremity.
- Monitor and treat for shock, maintain body temperature, and administer high-flow oxygen.

Spine Injuries

Signs and Symptoms

- Constant or intermittent pain along the spinal column or extremities
- Obvious deformity
- Numbness, weakness, tingling in the extremities
- Soft-tissue injuries in the spinal region
- Loss of sensation
- Paralysis
- Incontinence
- Head or neck injury
- Abdominal excursion

Management

- Open and maintain a patent airway with the jaw-thrust maneuver.
- Perform manual in-line stabilization to protect the cervical spine.
- Consider inserting an oropharyngeal airway.
- Have a suctioning unit available.
- Provide high-flow oxygen to the patient.
- Continuously monitor the patient's airway.
- Prepare the patient for transport according to the patient's position.
- Transport the patient to the appropriate trauma center.

Stroke

Signs and Symptoms

- Facial drooping
- Sudden weakness or numbness in the face, arm, leg, or one side of the body
- Loss of movement and sensation on one side of the body
- Decreased or absent movement in one or more extremities
- Lack of muscle coordination (ataxia)
- Sudden vision loss in one eye, blurred and double vision
- Difficulty swallowing
- Decreased level of responsiveness
- Speech disorders (dysphasia)
- Absence of speech
- Sudden and severe headache
- Sudden loss of balance or trouble walking
- Confusion
- Dizziness
- Weakness
- Combativeness
- Restlessness
- Tongue deviation
- Coma

Management

- Determine the time of symptom onset.
- Observe the patient's position and protect any affected extremities.
- Administer high-flow oxygen to the patient.
- Perform a field stroke test such as the Cincinnati Prehospital Stroke scale or Los Angeles Prehospital Stroke screen.
- Monitor vital signs every 5 minutes; watch for trends in blood pressure measurements.
- Transport the patient to a stroke specialty center. Do not delay transport.

Table 6 Summary of Adult CPR

	One Rescuer	Two Rescuers
Rate	100-120 per minute	100-120 per minute
Ratio	30:2	30:2
Depth	2-2.4"	2-2.4"
Hand Placement	Center of chest	Center of chest
Rescue Breathing	10-12 per minute (1 breath every 5-6 seconds)	10-12 per minute (1 breath every 5-6 seconds)
Airway Obstruction	**Conscious:** Determine if the airway is completely obstructed. Deliver abdominal thrusts until the foreign body is expelled or the patient becomes unconscious. **Unconscious:** Begin CPR. Each time the airway is opened, look for an object in the patient's mouth and remove it.	

Table 7 · Summary of Infant and Child CPR

	Infant	Child
Age	1 month–1 year	1 year to onset of puberty
Location of Pulse Check	Brachial artery	Carotid or femoral artery
Rate	100–120 per minute	100–120 per minute
Ratio	30:2 (1 rescuer) 15:2 (2 rescuers)	30:2 (1 rescuer) 15:2 (2 rescuers)
Depth	At least one third depth of chest (about 1.5")	At least one third depth of chest (about 2")
Hand Placement	2 fingers or 2 thumb encircling-hands technique	Heel of one or both hands
Rescue Breathing	12–20 per minute (1 breath every 3–5 seconds)	12–20 per minute (1 breath every 3–5 seconds)
Airway Obstruction	**Conscious:** Determine if the airway is obstructed. Deliver 5 back slaps and 5 chest thrusts. **Unconscious:** Begin CPR. Each time the airway is opened, look for an object in the patient's mouth and remove it.	**Conscious:** Determine if the airway is obstructed. Deliver abdominal thrusts until the foreign body is expelled. **Unconscious:** Begin CPR. Each time the airway is opened, look for an object in the patient's mouth and remove it.

Infants and Children: Special Situations

Tracheostomy Tube

- Maintain an open airway.
- Be prepared to suction the tube.
- **Place the patient in a position of comfort during transport.**

Mechanical Ventilator

- Enlist the aid of caregivers familiar with the unit.
- Provide ventilations with a bag-mask device if appropriate.

Central IV Lines

- If bleeding is noted from the site, **apply direct pressure over the site** using a sterile dressing and a gloved hand. Provide immediate transport to the hospital.

Gastrostomy Tube

- Have a suction unit readily available to clear the patient's airway as needed.
- Patients who have difficulty breathing should be transported either sitting or lying on the right side with the head elevated 30° to prevent the contents of the stomach from entering the lungs.
- Give supplemental oxygen if the patient has any difficulty breathing.
- Monitor the patient for changes in level of consciousness, especially if the patient is diabetic, because these individuals may quickly become hypoglycemic.

Shunt

- If the shunt malfunctions, pressure inside the patient's skull will rise, causing altered mental status.
- Watch for changes in level of consciousness or ventilation difficulties.
- **The patient may stop breathing.** Provide artificial ventilations if necessary.

Table 8 Vital Signs Chart: Infants and Children

Age	Temperature (°F)	Pulse Rate	Respiratory Rate	Blood Pressure (Systolic, mm Hg)
Neonate (0 to 1 month)	98 to 100	90 to 180	30 to 60	50 to 70
Infant (1 month to 1 year)	96.8 to 99.6	100 to 160	25 to 50	70 to 95
Toddler (1 to 3 years)	96.8 to 99.6	90 to 150	20 to 30	80 to 100
Preschool-age (3 to 6 years)	98.6	80 to 140	20 to 25	80 to 100
School-age (6 to 12 years)	98.6	70 to 120	15 to 20	80 to 110
Adolescent (12 to 18 years)	98.6	60 to 100	12 to 20	90 to 110
Early adult (19 to 40 years)	98.6	60 to 100	12 to 20	90 to 140
Middle adult (41 to 60 years)	98.6	60 to 100	12 to 20	90 to 140
Late adult (61 and older)	98.6	Depends on health	Depends on health	Depends on health

Age Cutoff for Blood Pressure and Capillary Refill

- Check blood pressure in children older than 3 years of age.
- Check capillary refill in infants and children younger than 6 years of age.

Rapid Formula: Lower Limits of Blood Pressure for Pediatric Patients (Age 1 to 10)

70 + (2 × child's age in years) = systolic blood pressure

Use an appropriate-size blood pressure cuff.

Blood Pressure for Patients in Extremely Serious Condition

Table 9 Systolic Blood Pressures Indicating an Extremely Serious Condition

Age	Systolic Blood Pressure (mm Hg)
Infant to 5 years	Less than 50
5 to 12 years	Less than 60
Teenager	Less than 70

Medications Carried in the Ambulance

Oxygen • Oral glucose • Activated charcoal • Epinephrine • Aspirin

Medications Carried by the Patient

Epinephrine auto-injector • Nitroglycerin • Metered-dose inhaler medications

General Guidelines for Medication Administration

- Obtain an online or off-line order from medical control.
- Verify the proper medication and prescription.
- Verify the form, dose, and route of the medication.
- Check the expiration date and condition of the medication.
- Reassess the patient's vital signs, especially pulse rate and blood pressure, at least every 5 minutes or as the patient's condition changes.
- Document the care given to the patient.
- After administering the medication, reassess and document the patient's condition:
  - Level of consciousness
  - Airway
  - Pulse, breathing, skin condition, blood pressure
  - Change in or relief of patient complaints
  - Side effects of medication
  - Improvement or deterioration of patient's condition

Six Rights of Medication Administration

- Right patient
- Right medication
- Right dose
- Right route
- Right time
- Right documentation

Common Drug Categories

Table 10 Selected Drug Categories	
Analgesic	Provides pain relief
Antiarrhythmic	Controls abnormal heart rhythms (such as rapid or slow rates, extra beats)
Antidiabetic	Helps patient maintain blood glucose level
Antihypertensive	Controls high blood pressure
Bronchodilator	Relaxes smooth muscle of the bronchial tubes, making breathing easier

Oxygen

Oxygen Flow Rates for the EMT

Nonrebreathing mask: 10 to 15 L/min (Reservoir bag should not collapse when the patient inhales.)

Nasal cannula: 2 to 6 L/min (A nasal cannula should be used only if the patient will not tolerate a nonrebreathing mask.)

Consult local protocols regarding oxygen administration to patients with COPD or emphysema.

Mouth-to-mask or bag-mask device: 15 L/min

Common Oxygen Tank Capacities

D = 350 liters
Super D = 500 liters
E = 625 liters
M = 3,000 liters
G = 5,300 liters
H, A, K = 6,900 liters

Pressure in a full tank: approximately 2,000 psi

Oxygen Cylinder Hydrostatic Testing

Steel: every 5 years
Aluminum: every 5 years

Duration of Oxygen Flow Formula

$$\frac{\text{Gauge pressure (psi)} - 200 \text{ psi (safe residual)} \times \text{cylinder constant}}{\text{Flow rate (L/min)}} = \text{Duration of flow (min)}$$

Cylinder Size	A	D	E	G	H	K	M
Constant	3.14	0.16	0.28	2.41	3.14	3.14	1.56

Example: A "D" cylinder with 1,800 psi flowing at 15 L/min would last 17 minutes (1,800 − 200 = 1,600, × the constant 0.16 = 256, ÷15 = 17.07)

◻ Oral Glucose

Indications

Patient presents with an altered mental status and has a known history of diabetes controlled by medication.

Contraindications

Unresponsive; unable to swallow

Actions

Increases blood glucose level

Side Effects

When given properly, oral glucose does not produce any side effects. If the patient does not have a gag reflex, the glucose may be aspirated.

Dosage

- Adult: one tube
- Child: one tube (Always follow the local protocol.)

Suggested Steps for Administration

- **The patient must be conscious and able to swallow.**
- Consult medical control for authorization.
- Administer glucose between the patient's cheek and gums.

If a Tongue Depressor Is Used:

- Place glucose on the bottom third of the tongue depressor.
- Place the tongue depressor between the patient's cheek and gums with gel toward the cheek.
- Allow the gel to dissolve or instruct the patient to swallow it.

Always Consider Other Possible Causes of Altered Mental Status

- Head trauma
- Seizures
- Poisoning
- Infection
- Hypoxia (decreased oxygen level)
- Hypothermia or hyperthermia
- Intoxication (other medical problems may still be present)

Activated Charcoal

Indications

Poisoning by ingestion (by mouth)

Contraindications

Altered mental status; unable to swallow; ingestion of acids or alkalis

Activated charcoal should not be administered if the patient ingested hydrocarbons, corrosives, caustics, petroleum substances, or metals

Actions

Activated charcoal binds to certain poisons, preventing them from being absorbed into the body as they pass through the digestive tract. **Note:** Brands of activated charcoal differ; some bind much more poison than others. Consult your medical director about which brand to use.

Side Effects

Vomiting, particularly if the patient has ingested a poison that causes nausea (repeat the dose once if the patient vomits); black stools

Dosage

- Adult: 1 to 2 g/kg of body weight
  Usual adult dose: 25–50 g
- Child and infant: 1 g/kg of body weight
  Usual infant and child dose: 12.5–25 g

Suggested Steps for Administration

- Shake the container thoroughly to mix the medication.
- Pour the liquid into a container (preferably with a lid and straw to hide the activated charcoal from the view of the patient).
- Have the patient drink the medication.

Additional Notes

- The patient may need to be persuaded to drink the medication because it looks like mud.
- If the patient takes a long time to drink the medication, shake or stir the medication again.
- Repeat the dose once if the patient vomits.
- Because vomiting is likely and the emesis can be quite messy, have a large container readily available into which the patient can vomit.
- The medication is available premixed in water.
- Avoid the use of powders in the field

Indications of Possible Poison Ingestion

- Burns, swelling, discoloration, or stains around the mouth
- Dry mouth or excessive salivation
- Pain in the mouth or throat and/or when swallowing
- Unusual mouth odors
- Abdominal pain, cramping, tenderness, and/or distention
- Nausea, vomiting, and/or diarrhea
- Altered mental status
- Altered vital signs

Examples of Compounds Bound by Activated Charcoal

Acetaminophen (Tylenol)

Alcohol

Amphetamines

Aspirin

Barbiturates

Cocaine

Darvon

Digitalis

Digitoxin

Digoxin

Ibuprofen

Imipramine

Iodine

Ipecac

Malathion

Morphine

Narcotics

Nortriptyline

Opium

Parathion

Penicillin

Phenol

Phenothiazines

Propoxyphene

Quinine

Salicylates

Strychnine

Tricyclic antidepressants

Epinephrine Auto-Injector

Indications

The patient must meet the following three criteria:

- The patient must exhibit the assessment findings of an allergic reaction (primarily those of a severe reaction, including respiratory distress and/or signs and symptoms of shock).
- Medication must be prescribed for this patient.
- Medical control must authorize use for this patient.

Contraindications

None, when used in a life-threatening situation

Actions

Dilates the bronchioles; constricts blood vessels

Side Effects

Increased pulse rate; pallor; dizziness; chest pain; headache; nausea; vomiting; excitability; anxiousness

Dosage

- **Adult:** one adult auto-injector (0.3 mg)
- **Child and infant:** one infant/child auto-injector (0.15 mg)

Suggested Steps for Administration

- Obtain the patient's prescribed auto-injector.
- If able to see the medication, do not use the auto-injector if it is discolored.
- Remove the safety cap.
- If possible, remove clothing from the injection site (may administer medication through thin clothing if necessary).
- If possible, wipe the injection site with alcohol.
- Place the tip of the injector against the lateral portion of the patient's thigh midway between the waist and knee (may also inject in fleshy portion of the patient's upper arm).
- Push firmly until the injector activates.

- Hold the injector in place 10 seconds or until the medication is injected.
- Massage the site to enhance absorption.
- Dispose of the auto-injector in the proper biohazard container.

Additional Notes

- Take the auto-injector with the patient to the hospital.
- Medical control may order a second dose.
- Some patients also carry oral antihistamines. If present, consult medical control concerning their use.

Common Signs and Symptoms of an Allergic Reaction

Respiratory

- Wheezing, stridor, or cough
- Tight feeling in the throat or chest
- Rapid breathing

Skin

- Itching
- Flushed (red) skin
- Hives
- Swelling (especially of the face, neck, tongue, hands, and/or feet)

Cardiac

- Increased pulse
- Decreased blood pressure

Other

- Runny nose
- Itchy, watery eyes
- Headache
- Nausea and/or vomiting
- Altered mental status

Nitroglycerin

Indications

Patient must meet the following three criteria:

- The patient exhibits signs and symptoms of chest pain.
- Medication must be prescribed for this patient.
- Medical control must authorize use for this patient.

Contraindications

- Hypotension or systolic blood pressure of less than 100 mm Hg
- Head injury
- Patient is an infant or child
- Patient has already reached maximum prescribed dose for medication prior to EMT arrival
- Patient is taking an erectile dysfunction drug such as Viagra (Consult medical control. Nitroglycerin may cause a serious drop in this patient's blood pressure.)

Actions

Dilates coronary arteries, increasing blood flow and oxygen supply to heart muscle; relaxes smooth muscle of blood vessel walls; decreases workload of heart

Side Effects

Hypotension; headache; pulse rate changes

Dosage

- Adult: one dose, repeated in 5 minutes if:
  - No relief of pain, and
  - Blood pressure remains greater than 100 mm Hg systolic, and
  - Medical control authorizes additional doses (up to a maximum of 3 doses)
- Child and infant: not for children and infants

Suggested Steps for Administration

- The patient's blood pressure must be above 100 mm Hg systolic.
- Check the expiration date of the medication. If nitroglycerin is older than 6 months, it may have lost its potency. (**If the prescription is old, the EMT may ask if the patient has a newer bottle.**)
- Ask the patient if he or she has already taken any, and if so, how many taken, when taken, and what effects the medication had on the patient.

If Medical Control Orders Administration

- Wear gloves. Nitroglycerin can be absorbed through the skin and can affect the EMT in the same way as it does the patient.
- Have the patient lift the tongue, and place the tablet or spray dose under the tongue.
- If nitroglycerin is a tablet, advise the patient to close the mouth and not to chew or swallow until the tablet dissolves and is absorbed.
- **Recheck the patient's blood pressure within 5 minutes.**

Additional Notes

- Continually monitor the patient's blood pressure.
- **If the blood pressure drops or the patient feels faint, lay the patient down.**
- Ask the patient about pain relief.
- Ask the patient whether the medication burned under the tongue or caused a headache.
- Consult medical control before readministering nitroglycerin.

If a patient who must be defibrillated is wearing a nitroglycerin patch on the chest, remove the nitroglycerin patch before defibrillating.

◼ Prescribed Inhaler

Indications

Patient must meet all the following criteria:

- The patient must exhibit signs and symptoms of a respiratory emergency (wheezing may be heard when listening to breath sounds).
- The patient must have a physician-prescribed inhaler.
- Medical control may need to give authorization for use.

Contraindications

- Patient is unable to use device
- Inhaler is not prescribed for the patient
- Hypersensitivity
- Tachycardia
- Myocardial infarction
- Medical control does not grant permission for use
- Patient has already reached maximum prescribed dose for medication prior to EMT arrival

Actions

Relaxes smooth muscles in the bronchial tubes, causing them to dilate and making breathing easier

Side Effects

Increased pulse rate; tremors; nervousness

Dosage

Adult and child: Maximum number of inhalations varies. Total number is based on orders from medical control or orders from the patient's physician (consult with the patient).

Table 11 Common Inhaler Names	
Generic Name	**Trade Name**
albuterol	Proventil, Ventolin
bitolterol mesylate	Tornalate
isoetharine	Bronkometer, Bronkosol
metaproterenol	Alupent, Metaprel
salmeterol xinafoate	Serevent

Suggested Steps for Administration

- Ask if the patient has already taken any doses and compare with the prescribed dose.
- Ensure that the inhaler is at room temperature or warmer.
- If a spacer device is available, place it on the inhaler.
- Stop administering supplemental oxygen and remove any mask from the patient.
- Have the patient exhale deeply.
- Tell the patient to put the mouthpiece in his or her mouth and make a seal with the lips.
- Instruct the patient to inhale slowly and deeply. Depress the patient's inhaler canister to deliver medication while the patient is inhaling.
- Have the patient hold his or her breath for as long as comfortably possible.
- Place the patient back on oxygen.

Additional Notes

- Medical control may order additional doses.
- If an over-the-counter inhaler is present, the EMT will not likely assist the patient in using it.

Special Notes About Children With Asthma

- When experiencing bronchospasm associated with asthma, children will often cough rather than wheeze.
- Look for retractions, use of accessory muscles (eg, neck, back, and abdominal muscles), and/or nasal flaring as indications of respiratory distress.

Aspirin

Indications

Patient presents with signs and symptoms indicative of a heart attack

Contraindications

Hypersensitivity to aspirin; preexisting liver damage; bleeding disorders; asthma

Actions

Inhibits platelet aggregation (clumping)

Side Effects

Nausea; vomiting; stomach pain; bleeding; allergic reaction

Dosage

Adult:160–325 mg (two to four 81-mg "baby" aspirin)

Suggested Steps for Administration

- **Patient must be conscious and able to chew tablets.**
- Baby aspirin will be easier for the patient to chew. Baby aspirin contains 81 mg of aspirin.
- Consult medical control for authorization where appropriate.

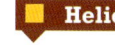

Radio Report Outline

Sample Radio Communication Patient Care Report Outline

(See Hospital Phone Number/Radio Channel List on Page 113)

- Unit identity and level of care
- Estimated time of arrival
- Patient's age and gender
- Chief complaint
- Brief, pertinent history of the present illness or injury
- Pertinent past medical history
- Mental status
- Baseline vital signs
- Pertinent findings of the physical examination
- Description of the emergency medical care given
- Patient's response to the care given

Note: The above list contains the essential elements in the order they should be given as outlined in the *EMT National Standard Curriculum*.

Helicopter Landing Zone Guidelines

- Ideally the area will be 100 ft by 100 ft in size (requirements may vary based on helicopter).
- The landing area should be clear of poles, trees, power lines, pedestrians/spectators, and any other obstacles.
- Find a firm, smooth surface clear of loose debris, overhead wires, and tall or leaning trees.
- Mark the corners of the landing zone with weighted cones or position emergency vehicles at the corners of the landing zone with the headlights facing inward to form an X.
- When it is dark, direct any illumination toward the landing spot, not at the approaching helicopter.
- Advise the pilot of obstructions, wires, poles, and trees.

- Do not approach the helicopter unless instructed to do so by the crew.
- Always approach and depart the helicopter from the front. If it is on a slope, approach and depart only from the down-slope side.
- Never raise anything above your head around the helicopter.
- Smoking, open lights, flames, and running are never permitted within 50 ft of the helicopter.
- **See page 112 for Air Medical Service phone number.**

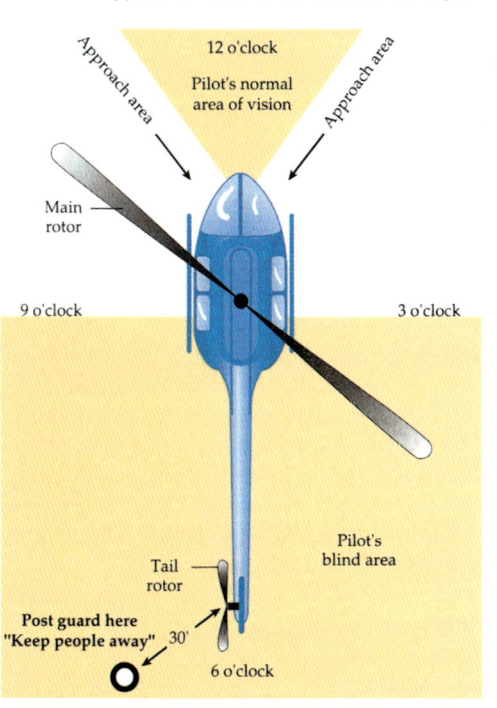

Approach routes for air medical helicopter

12 o'clock

Pilot's normal area of vision

Approach area

Approach area

Main rotor

9 o'clock

3 o'clock

Pilot's blind area

Tail rotor

Post guard here "Keep people away" 30'

6 o'clock

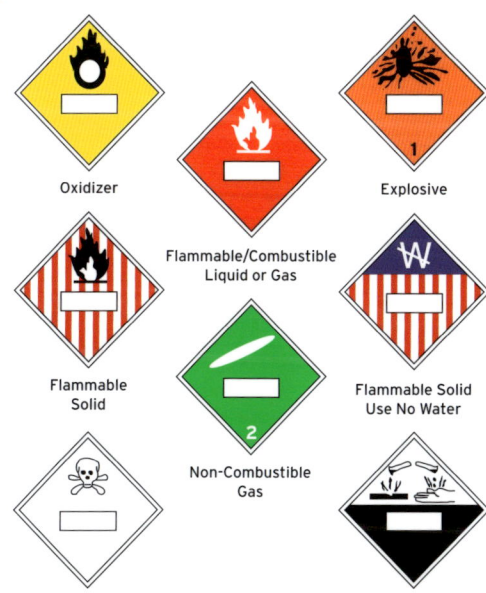

Oxidizer

Flammable/Combustible
Liquid or Gas

Explosive

Flammable
Solid

Non-Combustible
Gas

Flammable Solid
Use No Water

Poison

Corrosive

DOT Class		
1 Explosive	4 Solid	7 Radioactive
2 Gas	5 Oxidizer	8 Corrosive
3 Liquid	6 Poison	9 Miscellaneous Dangerous Goods

Modified from U.S. Department of Transportation.

Medical Group Supervisor

- Receive the appointment from the **Incident Commander or Operations Section Chief**.
- Don a command vest if available.
- Perform an assessment of the scene.
  - Assess the scene for hazards.
  - Keep the following priorities in mind: safety, incident stabilization, and preservation of property and the environment.
  - Determine which resources are needed.
- Request additional units and resources.
- Have communication center notify area hospitals that a mass-casualty incident (MCI) exists.
- **Assign a Triage Unit Leader, Treatment Unit Leader, and Transportation Unit Leader. Assign a Medical Supply Coordinator if needed. Determine if a Staging Area Manager has been assigned by Operations.**
- Determine if it is safe to begin operations.
- Use **tactical worksheets**, **status boards**, and/or **checklists** if available.
- Coordinate all EMS operations during the incident. Consult with other command personnel as needed for updates.
- Request law enforcement and coroner involvement as needed.
- Act as liaison with other medical support agencies.
- Assign and reassign personnel as necessary.
- Reevaluate the need for additional units and equipment.

Model Incident Command Structure for Mass-Casualty Incidents

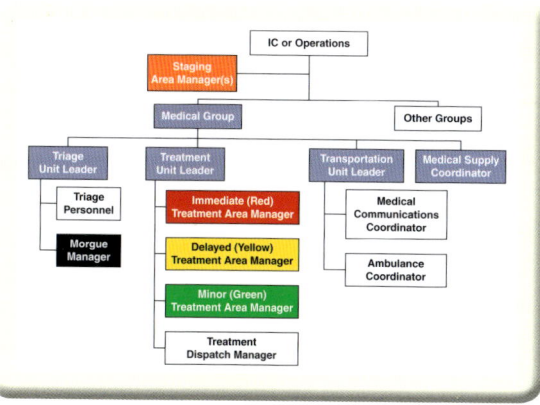

Triage Unit Leader

NO TREATMENT IS TO BE DONE IN THE TRIAGE AREA. Possible exceptions: rapid correction of life-threatening problems (eg, open airway, rapid bleeding control, or administering auto-injector antidotes).

- Obtain a briefing from the **Medical Group Supervisor**.
- Obtain **triage supplies** (ie, triage tags, ribbons).
- Don a **command vest** if available.
- Determine if patients will be **triaged where they are found** or taken to a **triage area**.
- Determine the equipment and personnel needs of the **Triage Unit**. Request same from the **Medical Group Supervisor**.
- Maintain close coordination with the **Treatment Unit** and the **Extrication Group**.
- Coordinate personnel assigned to the **Triage Unit**.
- Distribute triage tags or ribbons to support personnel as appropriate.
- Begin triage operations.
- Advise the **Treatment Unit Leader** and **Medical Group Supervisor** of the approximate number of patients as soon as possible.
- Coordinate the transfer of patients to the **Treatment Area** based on priority.
- Request personnel and equipment as needed to transfer patients to the **Treatment Area**.
- Assign a **Morgue Manager** if needed.
- Have all areas around the MCI scene checked for walk-aways, potential patients, ejected patients, and other casualties.
- Advise the **Treatment Unit Leader and Medical Group Supervisor** when initial triaging and tagging operations are complete.
- Begin relieving or reducing staff as necessary.
- Report to the **Medical Group Supervisor** for reassignment on completion of tasks.

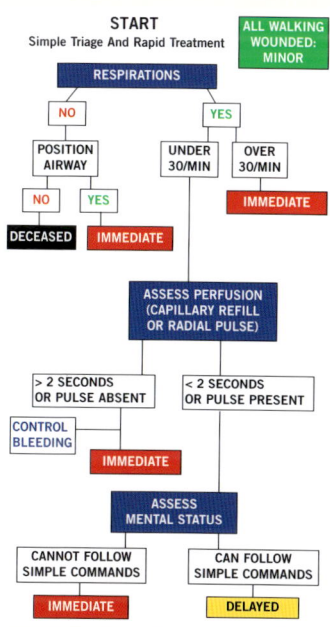

START
Simple Triage And Rapid Treatment

ALL WALKING WOUNDED: MINOR

RESPIRATIONS
- NO → POSITION AIRWAY
  - NO → DECEASED
  - YES → IMMEDIATE
- YES
  - UNDER 30/MIN
  - OVER 30/MIN → IMMEDIATE

ASSESS PERFUSION (CAPILLARY REFILL OR RADIAL PULSE)
- > 2 SECONDS OR PULSE ABSENT → CONTROL BLEEDING / IMMEDIATE
- < 2 SECONDS OR PULSE PRESENT

ASSESS MENTAL STATUS
- CANNOT FOLLOW SIMPLE COMMANDS → IMMEDIATE
- CAN FOLLOW SIMPLE COMMANDS → DELAYED

Used with permission of Hoag Memorial Hospital Presbyterian and the Newport Beach Fire Department.

SALT Triage System

SALT = Sort – Assess – Lifesaving Interventions – Treatment and/or Transport

Step 1 – Sort: Begins with a **global sorting** of patients and prioritize them for individual assessment. *All patients should eventually receive an individual assessment.*

Ask Ambulatory patients to walk to a designated area. As a group they are assessed third **(last priority)**.

Ask those who remain to wave (ie, follow a command) and also observe for purposeful movements. Those who make purposeful movements are assessed second.

Those who do not move (ie, are still) and those with obvious life threats should be assessed first since they are the most likely to need lifesaving interventions.

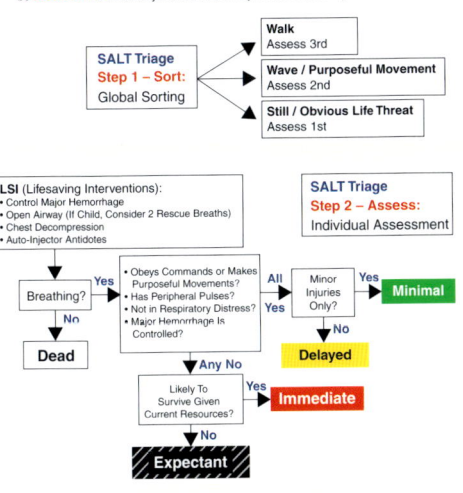

Reproduced from E.B. Lerner, et al., Mass Casualty Triage: An Evaluation of the Data and Development of a Proposed National Guideline, *Disaster Medicine and Public Health Preparedness* 2(1): S25.

- Obtain a briefing from the **Medical Group Supervisor**.
- Don a **command vest** if available.
- Determine the equipment and personnel needs of the **Treatment Unit**. Request same from the **Medical Group Supervisor**.
- The **Treatment Unit Leader** should **NOT** become involved in physical tasks.
- Coordinate personnel assigned to the **Treatment Unit**.
- Establish a primary **Treatment Area**.
- Think big with room to grow: The Treatment Area must be capable of accommodating large numbers of patients and equipment.
- Consider weather, safety, and hazardous materials.
- The Treatment Area must be readily accessible.
- Designate an **Entrance** and an **Exit** to the Treatment Area.
- Divide the Treatment Area into **four distinct** and well-marked sections. Use appropriate colored flags, tarps and/or barricade tape.
  - **Red**: first priority (critical problems)
  - **Yellow**: second priority (moderate problems)
  - **Green**: third priority (minor problems)
  - **Black**: morgue
- **Do not establish the Black area (morgue) near living victims.** (Fatalities will generally not be moved from the actual scene until later, so this area will initially mainly receive only patients who die in the Treatment Area.)
- Coordinate with law enforcement to provide security for fatalities.

- Designate a secondary Treatment Area as an alternative should the primary Treatment Area become unusable.
- Inform the **Triage Unit Leader** and **Medical Group Supervisor** of the primary and secondary Treatment Area locations.
- Consider assigning a **Treatment Dispatch Manager** to coordinate the transportation of patients.
- Consider assigning **Area Managers** for the Red, Yellow, and Green areas.
- Assign personnel to Treatment Areas based on their medical capabilities.
- Coordinate with the **Triage Unit Leader** regarding movement of patients from the field to the Treatment Area.
- Reassess and retriage patients on arrival at the Treatment Area.
- Send patients to appropriate sections of the Treatment Area.
- Place patients who are in greatest need of transport near Treatment Area exits.
- Continually reassess supplies on hand or needed, and request additional supplies if necessary (consider MCI units/trailers if available).
- Complete a **Treatment Sector Log** as patients enter and leave the Treatment Area.
- Notify the **Transportation Unit Leader** if a patient may need special care (eg, burn, brain injury, surgery) that only certain area hospitals can provide. Evacuate patients by priority.
- Begin relieving or reducing staff as necessary.
- Remain in the Treatment Area until reassigned or until all patients have been transported.
- Report to the **Medical Group Supervisor** for reassignment on completion of tasks.

Only unit to communicate with hospital

- Obtain a briefing from the **Medical Group Supervisor**.
- Don a **command vest** if available.
- Determine equipment and personnel needs of the **Transportation Unit**.
- Coordinate personnel assigned to the **Transportation Unit**.
- The **Transportation Unit Leader** should **NOT** become involved in physical tasks.
- Consider appointing a **Medical Communications Coordinator** and **a Ground Ambulance Coordinator**. **Operations** may assign an **Air Operations Branch Director** for coordinating helicopters.
- Provide and coordinate patient transport.
- Communicate with area hospitals (**refer to the Hospital Telephone Number section on page 113**).
- **Be specific but brief**:
  - Relay information about the incident to hospitals as needed.
  - Ascertain each hospital's capabilities and the number of emergency room and surgical cases that can be handled.
  - Inform hospitals of the number of patients to expect and their conditions.
- Establish some type of **Hospital Capability and Patient Tally Sheet** to use as a reference to avoid overloading individual hospitals.
- Consult with the **Treatment Dispatch Manager** and establish an **Ambulance Loading Zone**. This zone should have separate Entrance and Exit routes.

- Consult with the **Air Operations Branch Director** to establish the location of the **Landing Zone** for helicopters.
- Advise the **Staging Area Manager** of the locations of the **Ambulance Loading Zone** and **Landing Zone**, as well as the best routes for access.
- Request ambulances from the **Staging Area Manager** as needed. Advise which level of care is required (ie, **EMT**, **AEMT**, **Paramedic**).
- Have the **Medical Communications Coordinator**, with possible assistance from **Transport Recorders**, maintain a **Hospital Transportation Log** listing the following information:
  - **EMS transport unit**
  - **Number of patients in unit**
  - **Patient triage tag number and name if available**
  - **Patient condition**
  - **Hospital destination**
  - **Time when the EMS unit left the Loading Zone**
- If triage tags are used, make sure each tag is filled out properly. **Keep one corner or section of the tag**.
- Make sure the driver of each ambulance knows to which hospital to transport the patient and has directions to the hospital.
- Continuously update the **Hospital Capability and Patient Tally Sheet** as patients are transported. Tally totals at the conclusion of the incident.
- Advise hospitals:
  - **Which units are responding to their facility**
  - **The number of patients and general condition**
  - **ETA of ambulance to hospital**

  Note: If a **Medical Communications Coordinator** is assigned, he or she should handle this task. **Individual ambulances should not communicate directly with hospitals** (possible exception: if the patient condition deteriorates or medical consultation is needed).

- Consider requesting **buses** to transport Green (minor) patients.
- Begin relieving or reducing staff as necessary.
- Advise hospitals and the **Medical Group Supervisor** when the last patient is transported.
- Report to the **Medical Group Supervisor** for reassignment on completion of tasks.

Important Note on Establishing Helicopter Landing Zones at MCIs: Landing Zones should be located distant enough from the **Treatment Area** so as not to create problems related to rotor wash or excessive noise. An ambulance may be assigned to ferry patients from the **Treatment Area** to the **Loading Zone**.

Staging Area Manager

- The **Staging Area Manager** normally reports to the **Operations Section Chief**. In an MCI, it may be advantageous to have a separate area for ambulances within the staging area.
- Obtain a briefing from the **Medical Group Supervisor**.
- When determining the location of the **Staging Area**, consider these points:
  - The EMS Staging Area may need to be distinct from the Fire Staging Area, but may be in same general location.
  - Think big: The Staging Area must be capable of accommodating large numbers of ambulances.
  - Consider safety and hazardous materials.
  - The area must be readily accessible.
  - Designate an **Entrance** and an **Exit** to the Staging Area.
  - Consider dividing the Staging Area into **three distinct** and well-marked areas for **EMT**, **AEMT**, and **Paramedic units**.
- Consider the need for a secondary **Staging Area** as an alternative should the primary Staging Area become unusable.

- Proceed to the Staging Area.
- Don a **command vest** if available.
- **Identify** the Staging Area with a **flag** or **some other type of marker** if available.
- Determine the equipment and personnel needs of the **Staging Area**. Request same from **Operations**.
- Coordinate personnel assigned to the Staging Area.
- Maintain some type of **Staging Area Log** listing the following information:
  - Time each unit arrives and leaves the Staging Area
  - Number of personnel onboard
  - Special equipment available
  - Radio communications capability
- Ascertain from the **Ground Ambulance Coordinator** the location of the Ambulance Loading Zone and the best route from the Staging Area to the Loading Zone.
- Coordinate with the **Ground Ambulance Coordinator** on requests for ambulances.
- Notify the **Ground Ambulance Coordinator** when the number of ambulances or a particular type of resource is at or near minimum reserve level.
- Provide briefings and other information to arriving EMS units as appropriate.
- Provide routing instructions for ambulances when they are sent to the Loading Zone.
- Send the proper number and types of units to the Loading Zone when requested by the **Ground Ambulance Coordinator**.
- Request maintenance/support services for staged units as needed.
- Remain at this post until reassigned or all patients have been transported.
- Report to the **Operations Section Chief** for reassignment on completion of tasks.

Key Items to Consider When Writing a Patient Care Report

Respiratory Distress/Shortness of Breath

- OPQRST
- Skin color (especially note cyanosis)
- Breath sounds (especially note the presence of wheezes, rales, or rhonchi)
- Use of accessory muscles; presence of retractions, nasal flaring, pursed lips
- Swelling in ankles (present or absent)
- Sharp pain (present or absent) with deep breath
- Jugular vein distention (present or absent)
- Ability to speak in full sentences
- Use of home breathing treatments and how many
- EMT interventions and effects (including assisting with use of prescribed inhaler)

Diabetic Emergency

- Level of consciousness
- OPQRST (especially note whether onset was rapid or gradual)
- Patient skin color (especially note if pale or flushed)
- Sweating (present or absent)
- Kussmaul respirations (rapid, deep breathing)
- Medications: Does the patient take insulin or oral diabetes medications?
- If diabetes medications taken, time of last insulin injection or when last pill was taken and dose
- Time when the patient last ate, or if the patient missed a meal or vomited after eating
- Recent patient blood glucose levels, if available

- Any unusual exercise or increased stress
- Ingestion of alcohol or other drugs
- EMT interventions and effects (including administration of oral glucose)

Chest Pain/Cardiac Problems

- OPQRST (especially note activity at time of onset; if pain is dull pressure or sharp; if pain radiates)
- Breath sounds (especially note rales and/or rhonchi)
- Sweating (present or absent)
- Nausea/vomiting (present or absent)
- Swelling in ankles (present or absent)
- Jugular vein distention (present or absent)
- EMT and/or patient interventions and effects (such as the use of aspirin and/or nitroglycerin)

Altered Level of Consciousness

- Describe the episode
- Describe the onset
- Note the duration of the episode
- Document any associated symptoms or signs
- Note evidence of diabetes (low blood glucose [hypoglycemia] or high blood glucose [hyperglycemia]), hypoxia, trauma (especially head injury), seizures, fever, poisoning/overdose, alcohol, hypothermia, or hyperthermia
- EMT interventions and effects

Poisoning/Overdose

- Substance involved
- Was incident accidental or intentional?
- Past history of suicide attempts
- Time when substance was ingested or patient was exposed
- Amount of substance involved

- Time period over which substance was ingested or patient was exposed
- Effects of substance on the patient (eg, decreased level of consciousness, nausea/vomiting/diarrhea, abdominal pain, burns around the mouth)
- Patient's weight
- Associated alcohol or drug ingestion
- EMT interventions and effects (including administration of activated charcoal)

Trauma

General:
- Type of incident
- Mechanism of injury
- Level of consciousness
- Estimated amount of external blood loss if present
- Was patient ambulatory following injury?
- **Spinal immobilization (thoroughly document)**
- Findings of the secondary assessment
- For extremity injuries: deformity, discoloration, circulation, motor, and sensory status

For head injuries also note:
- Any loss of consciousness, amnesia, or change in behavior
- Any seizure activity
- Blood or fluid coming from the ears and/or nose
- Discoloration around eyes or behind ears
- Nausea and/or vomiting

For vehicle crashes also note:
- Type of crash: rear-ended, head-on, side impact (T-bone), rollover
- Speed of vehicle(s)
- Description of vehicle damage (**take digital photos if indicated**)
- Patient's position in vehicle

- Was patient wearing safety belts (lap, shoulder, both)?
- Deployment of air bag/passive restraint system
- Was patient ejected?
- Was patient entrapped, and if so, length of extrication?

For gunshot or stab wounds also note:

- Number and location of wounds
- Type of weapon: If gun, note type (handgun, shotgun, rifle) and caliber. If knife, note length and type of blade, and knife angle at time of stabbing.
- Patient's position at time of injury
- Perpetrator's position at time of assault
- Presence or notification of law enforcement personnel

Allergic Reaction

- History of allergies
- Substance to which patient was exposed
- Method of exposure
- Effects of exposure (especially note tightness in throat or chest, swelling of face/neck/tongue, wheezing, itching, hives, flushed skin)
- Progression of effects
- EMT interventions and effects (including assisting with administration of epinephrine)

Environmental Emergency

- Source
- Type of environment (cold, heat)
- Duration of exposure to source
- General or local effects
- Loss of consciousness
- EMT interventions and effects

Childbirth/Obstetric Emergency

General:

- Last menstrual period and possibility of pregnancy
- Use of birth control and method
- Presence of bleeding or discharge
- Presence of abdominal pain, fever, or signs of shock

If patient is pregnant also note:

- Estimated due date
- Prenatal care received by the patient
- Previous number of pregnancies (gravida) and number carried to term (para)
- Is the patient having pain and/or contractions? (If so, note time started, duration, and frequency.)
- Has the patient's water broken? (If so, note when and what color.)
- Presence of crowning, prolapsed cord or limb, or breech presentation
- Does the patient have urge to push?
- Complications encountered with this or other pregnancies
- EMT interventions and effects

Bones of the Body

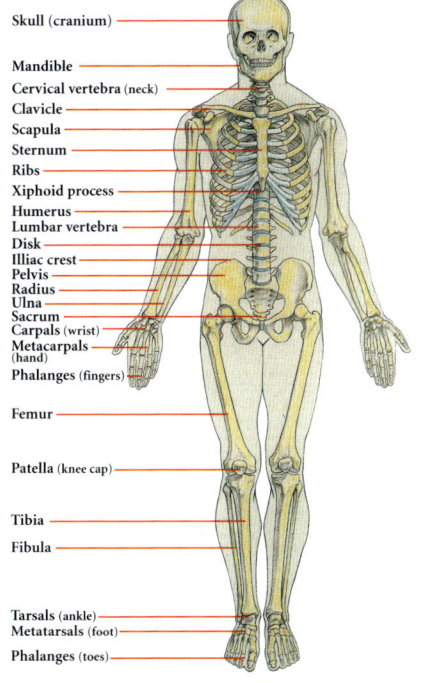

Skull (cranium)

Mandible
Cervical vertebra (neck)
Clavicle
Scapula
Sternum
Ribs
Xiphoid process
Humerus
Lumbar vertebra
Disk
Illiac crest
Pelvis
Radius
Ulna
Sacrum
Carpals (wrist)
Metacarpals (hand)
Phalanges (fingers)

Femur

Patella (knee cap)

Tibia

Fibula

Tarsals (ankle)
Metatarsals (foot)

Phalanges (toes)

A

abdomen
abrasion
abruptio placentae
abscess
allergy
amniotic
amphetamines
amputation
anaphylactic
anemia
aneurysm
angina
angulated
anoxia
antibiotic
antidepressant
aortic
apnea/apneic
appendicitis
arrhythmia
arteriosclerosis
arthritis
asphyxia
aspirate
assess

atrial
auscultation
avulsion
axillary

B

bacterial
barbiturates
belligerent
benign
bilateral
bile
biopsy
bowel
brachial
bronchial
bronchitis
bronchospasm
bursitis

C

cannula
capillary
cardiogenic
carotid
carpal
cartilage

cataracts
catheter
cephalic
cerebral
cervix
cesarean
chemotherapy
cholesterol
chronic
cirrhosis
coccyx
collapse
colon
colostomy
concussion
congenital
conjunctivitis
conscious
constipated
contagious
contusion
convulsion
coronary
croup
cyanotic

D

decerebrate
decorticate
defibrillate
defibrillator
dehydrated
delirium
deteriorate
diabetes
diaphoretic
diaphragm
diarrhea
diastolic
dislocation

E

ecchymosis
eclampsia
ectopic
edema
embolism
emphysema
epidermis
epiglottis
epiglottitis
epilepsy
epinephrine
epistaxis
esophagus
evisceration
extricated

F

fallopian
febrile
feces
femoral
femur
fetus
fibrillation
fibula
flail

G

gallbladder
gangrene
genital
geriatric
glaucoma
gonorrhea
grand mal

H

hallucination
hematoma
hemiplegia
hemophilia
hemoptysis
hemorrhage
hemorrhoid
hepatitis
hernia
herpes
hiatal
Hodgkin's
humerus
hypertension
hypertrophy
hyperventilate
hypochondriac
hypoglycemia
hypotension
hypothermia
hypovolemia
hypoxia
hysterectomy
hysteria

I

immobilize
inadequate
incision
incontinent
infarction
infectious
inflammation
ingestion
inhalation
insulin
intestine
intramuscular

intravenous
irritable
ischemia

J
jaundice
jugular

K
ketoacidosis
kidney

L
laceration
laryngectomy
larynx
lethargic
leukemia
ligament
lividity
lumbar
lymphoma

M
malaise
malignant
mandible
marijuana
mastectomy
measles
mediastinal

meningitis
menopause
menstrual
miscarriage
mitral
myocardial

N
narcotic
nasopharyngeal
nausea
neonatal
neurological
nocturnal

O
obstruction
occlusion
oriented
oropharyngeal
oropharynx
orthopaedic
orthopnea
ovaries
ovulation

P
palpation
pancreas
paralysis

paraplegia
parietal
paroxysmal
patella
pediatric
pelvic
penetrate
penicillin
perforated
perfusion
perineum
peripheral
peritoneum
peritonitis
persistent
petit mal
phalanges
pharynx
phlebitis
pituitary
placenta previa
pleural
pleurisy
pneumonia
pneumothorax
postictal
postpartum
preeclampsia

pregnant
prognosis
prolapsed
proximal
psychiatric
pulmonary
puncture

Q
quadriplegic

R
radial
radiate
rales
rectum
regurgitate
relief/relieve
renal
resistance
respiration
rhonchi
rhythm
rigor mortis

S
scapula
seizure
septum
sinus

sphygmomanometer
sputum
stenosis
sternum
stethoscope
stomach
stridor
subclavian
subcutaneous
sublingual
substernal
suicidal
superficial
symptom
syncope
syndrome
syphilis
syringe
systolic

T
temperature
tendon
thoracic
thrombosis
thyroid
tibia
tongue

tourniquet
toxemia
tracheostomy
tranquilizers
traumatic
Trendelenburg
tuberculosis
typhoid

U
ulcer
ulna
umbilical
unconscious
urinary
urine
uterus

V
vaginal
vascular
vasodilator
venous
ventilation
vomitus

W
wheeze

abd	abdomen
AIDS	acquired immuno deficiency syndrome
A & O	alert and oriented
ASA	aspirin
ASHD	arteriosclerotic heart disease
bid	twice a day
BM	bowel movement
BSA	body surface area
$\bar{c}$	with
CA	cancer
CABG	coronary artery bypass graft
CAD	coronary artery disease
CAP	capsule
CBC	complete blood count
CC	chief complaint
cc	cubic centimeter
CHF	congestive heart failure
CID	cervical immobilization device
cm	centimeter
CNS	central nervous system
CO	carbon monoxide
CO_2	carbon dioxide
COPD	chronic obstructive pulmonary disease
CSF	cerebrospinal fluid
CVA	cerebrovascular accident (stroke)
D/C	discontinue

DKA	diabetic ketoacidosis
DNR	do not resuscitate
DOB	date of birth
Dx	diagnosis
ET	endotracheal
ETA	estimated time of arrival
ETOH	ethyl alcohol
GCS	Glasgow Coma Scale
GI	gastrointestinal
GSW	gunshot wound
gt	drop
gtt	drops
GU	genitourinary
HIV	human immunodeficiency virus
HR	heart rate
hr (h)	hour
HTN	hypertension (high blood pressure)
Hx	history
IM	intramuscular
inj	injection; injury
IO	intraosseous
IV	intravenous
JVD	jugular vein distention
K^+	potassium
kg	kilogram
L	left
L	liter
LBB	long backboard

LLQ	left lower quadrant
LMP	last menstrual period
LOC	level of consciousness; loss of consciousness
lpm (LPM, L/min)	liters per minute
LUQ	left upper quadrant
m	meter
MCI	mass-casualty incident
mg	milligram
mcg	microgram
MI	myocardial infarction (heart attack)
min	minute; minimum
mL	milliliter
mm	millimeter
MOI	mechanism of injury
Na	sodium
NC	nasal cannula
neg	negative
NOI	nature of illness
NTG	nitroglycerin
N & V	nausea and vomiting
O_2	oxygen
OB	obstetrics
OBS	organic brain syndrome
OD	overdose; right eye
OS	left eye
OTC	over-the-counter
OU	both eyes

P̄	after
PAT	paroxysmal atrial tachycardia
PCN	penicillin
PE	physical exam or pulmonary embolism
PID	pelvic inflammatory disease
PO	by mouth
prn	as needed
Pt	patient
PVC	premature ventricular contraction
Px	physical examination
q	every
qAM	every morning
qd	every day
qh	every hour
q2h	every 2 hours
q3h	every 3 hours
q4h	every 4 hours
q6h	every 6 hours
q12h	every 12 hours
qid	4 times daily
qod	every other day
qPM	every night
R	right
RBC	red blood count or cell
RLQ	right lower quadrant
R/O	rule out
RUQ	right upper quadrant
Rx	medication or prescription

SC	subcutaneous
$\overline{s}$	without
sec (s)	second
SL	sublingual
SOB	shortness of breath
SQ	subcutaneous
tab	tablet
temp	temperature
TIA	transient ischemic attack
tid	three times daily
top	topical
Tx	treatment
UTI	urinary tract infection
VF	ventricular fibrillation
VS	vital signs
VT	ventricular tachycardia
WBC	white blood count or cell
W/	with
w/o	without
wk	week
wt	weight
yr	year

Prescription Medications

Trade names start with an uppercase letter and appear in **blue**. **Generic names** start with a lowercase letter and appear in **red**. The primary type of medical problem for which the medication is used is listed, and the type of medication is shown in parentheses when indicated. **Noting patients' medications can help the EMT determine which type of medical problems patients have even if they are unsure of their history or are unconscious.**

Abilify	bipolar disorder; schizophrenia
Accolate	asthma
Accupril	high blood pressure; congestive heart failure
acetaminophen with codeine	pain
Aciphex	gastric problems (antiulcer)
Actiq	pain (narcotic analgesic)
Actonel	osteoporosis
Actos	diabetes (oral antidiabetic)
acyclovir	viral infections (antiviral)
Adderall	attention-deficit/hyperactivity disorder
Adipex	weight loss
Advair	breathing problems
albuterol	breathing problems (bronchodilator)
Aldactazide	high blood pressure (diuretic/water pill)
Aldactone	congestive heart failure (diuretic/water pill)
Aldomet	high blood pressure

alendronate	osteoporosis
Alesse 28	birth control pills
Allegra	allergies (antihistamine)
Alli	weight loss
allopurinol	gout; kidney stones
alprazolam	anxiety; depression (sedative/antianxiety)
Altace	high blood pressure (ACE inhibitor)
Alupent	asthma; breathing problems (bronchodilator)
Amaryl	diabetes (oral antidiabetic)
Ambien	insomnia (hypnotic)
Amitiza	gastrointestinal problems
amitriptyline	depression (antidepressant)
amlodipine	high blood pressure; angina
amoxicillin	infection (antibiotic)
Amoxil	infection (antibiotic)
Anaprox	arthritis (anti-inflammatory)
Ansaid	arthritis (anti-inflammatory)
Antivert	dizziness; motion sickness (antivertigo)
Apresoline	high blood pressure (antihypertensive)
Aricept	Alzheimer disease
Artane	Parkinson disease (anti-Parkinson)
Arthrotec	arthritis (anti-inflammatory)
Asacol	ulcerative colitis (antibacterial)
Atarax	anxiety; behavioral disorders (sedative)

atenolol	high blood pressure; heart problems; angina (beta blocker)
Ativan	anxiety (sedative/antianxiety)
Atrovent	breathing problems (bronchodilator)
Augmentin	infection (antibiotic)
Avandamet	diabetes
Avandia	diabetes (oral antidiabetic)
Avapro	high blood pressure
Avodart	prostate enlargement
Axid	ulcers (antiulcer)
azithromycin	infection (antibiotic)
Azulfidine	ulcerative colitis (antibacterial)
Bactrim	infection (antibiotic)
Bactroban	impetigo (antibiotic)
benazepril	high blood pressure; congestive heart failure
Benicar	high blood pressure
Bentyl	irritable bowel syndrome (anticholinergic)
benzonatate	cough (antitussive)
Biaxin	infection (antibiotic)
bisoprolol	high blood pressure (diuretic)
Boniva	osteoporosis
Brethine	asthma; breathing problems (bronchodilator)
Bumex	edema; congestive heart failure (diuretic)

bupropion	depression; smoking cessation
BuSpar	anxiety (antianxiety)
buspirone	anxiety (antianxiety)
Byetta	diabetes
Caduet	high blood pressure
Calan	angina; high blood pressure; rapid heart rate
Capoten	high blood pressure; congestive heart failure
captopril	high blood pressure; congestive heart failure
Carafate	ulcers (antiulcer)
carbamazepine	seizure disorder (anticonvulsant)
Cardizem	heart problems; angina (coronary vasodilator)
Cardura	high blood pressure (alpha blocker)
carisoprodol	muscle spasms (muscle relaxant)
Cartia	angina; heart problems (calcium-channel blocker)
carvedilol	high blood pressure
Catapres	high blood pressure (antihypertensive)
Ceclor	infection (antibiotic)
cefaclor	infection (antibiotic)
cefdinir	infection (antibiotic)
cefixime	infection (antibiotic)
cefprozil	infection (antibiotic)
Ceftin	infection (antibiotic)

cefuroxime	infection (antibiotic)
Cefzil	infection (antibiotic)
Celebrex	arthritis (anti-inflammatory)
Celexa	depression (antidepressant)
cephalexin	infection (antibiotic)
cetirizine	antihistamine
Chantix	smoking cessation
Cialis	erectile dysfunction
Ciloxin	infection (antibiotic)
cimetidine	ulcers; gastric problems (antiulcer)
Cipro	infection (antibiotic)
citalopram	depression
Clarinex	allergies (antihistamine)
Claritin	allergies (antihistamine)
clarithromycin	infection (antibiotic)
clindamycin	infection (antibiotic)
Clinoril	arthritis pain (anti-inflammatory)
clonazepam	seizure disorder (anticonvulsant)
clonidine	high blood pressure (antihypertensive)
clopidogrel	antiplatelet
clotrimazole	fungal infection (antifungal)
Colestid	high cholesterol (cholesterol lowering agent)
Combivent	breathing problems (bronchodilator)
Compazine	nausea (antiemetic)
Concerta	attention-deficit/hyperactivity disorder

Coreg	high blood pressure; heart problems
Corgard	heart problems; angina (beta blocker)
Cotrim	infection (anti-infective)
Coumadin	blood clots (blood thinner)
Cozaar	high blood pressure
Crestor	high cholesterol
cyclobenzaprine	muscle spasms (muscle relaxant)
Cymbalta	depression
Darvocet-N	pain management (narcotic analgesic)
Daypro	arthritis (anti-inflammatory)
Deltasone	severe inflammation (anti-inflammatory)
Demadex	edema; congestive heart failure (diuretic)
Demerol	pain (narcotic analgesic)
Depakote	seizure disorder (anticonvulsant)
Desyrel	depression (antidepressant)
Detrol	overactive bladder
Dexedrine	narcolepsy; attention-deficit disorder
dexmethylphenidate	attention-deficit/hyperactivity disorder
DiaBeta	diabetes (oral antidiabetic)
Diabinese	diabetes (oral antidiabetic)
diazepam	anxiety (antianxiety)
diclofenac	inflammation (anti-inflammatory)
Diflucan	fungal infection (antifungal)
Digitek	heart problems

digoxin	heart problems
Dilantin	seizure disorder (anticonvulsant)
diltiazem	heart problems; angina (coronary vasodilator)
Diovan	high blood pressure (antihypertensive)
Dipentum	ulcerative colitis
Diprivan	anesthetic
dipyridamole	thromboembolism
Ditropan	bladder problems (antispasmodic)
Donnatal	irritable bowel syndrome (anticholinergic)
doxazosin	hypertension; prostate problems
doxycycline	infection (antibiotic)
Duricef	infection (antibiotic)
Dyazide	high blood pressure; edema (diuretic)
DynaCirc	high blood pressure
E.E.S.	infection (antibiotic)
Effexor	depression (antidepressant)
Elavil	depression (antidepressant)
Eldepryl	Parkinson disease (anti-Parkinson)
Elocon	dermatologic problems
Emend	nausea (antiemetic)
enalapril	high blood pressure; heart failure
Enbrel	rheumatoid arthritis
E-Mycin	infection (antibiotic)
Entex	cough and congestion (expectorant)

Ery-Tab	infection (antibiotic)
erythromycin	infection (antibiotic)
escitalopram	depression
Esidrix	high blood pressure (diuretic/water pill)
Eskalith	behavioral disorders (antimanic)
Estrace	estrogen therapy
Estraderm	estrogen therapy
estradiol	menopause; gynecologic problems
etodolac	arthritis; pain (anti-inflammatory)
Evista	osteoporosis
famotidine	ulcers; gastric problems (antiulcer)
Feldene	arthritis (anti-inflammatory)
finasteride	prostate enlargement
Fiorinal	pain management (non-narcotic analgesic)
Flagyl	infections (antibacterial)
Flexeril	muscle spasms (muscle relaxant)
flexofenadine	antihistamine
Flomax	enlarged prostate (alpha blocker)
Flonase	allergies
Flovent	breathing problems
Floxin	infection (antibiotic)
fluconazole	fungal infection
fluoxetine	depression (antidepressant)
flurbiprofen	inflammation (anti-inflammatory)
folic acid	anemia

Fosamax	osteoporosis
fosinopril	osteoporosis
furosemide	congestive heart failure (diuretic/water pill)
gabapentin	seizures
Gabitril	seizure disorder (antiseizure)
Gantrisin	infection (antibiotic)
gemfibrozil	high cholesterol (cholesterol lowering agent)
Geodon	antipsychotic
glimepiride	diabetes (hyperglycemia)
glipizide	diabetes (oral antidiabetic)
Glucophage	diabetes (oral antidiabetic)
Glucotrol	diabetes (oral antidiabetic)
Glucovance	diabetes (oral antidiabetic)
glyburide	diabetes (oral hypoglycemic)
Glycolax	constipation
granisetron	nausea
guaifenesin	cough and congestion (expectorant)
Halcion	insomnia (hypnotic/sedative)
Haldol	psychotic disorders (antipsychotic)
HCTZ	high blood pressure (diuretic/water pill)
Humira	rheumatoid arthritis
Humulin	diabetes (insulin)
hydrochlorothiazide	high blood pressure (diuretic)
hydrocodone	cough; pain (narcotic)

HydroDiuril	high blood pressure (diuretic/water pill)
hydroxyzine	anxiety; behavioral disorders (sedative)
Hygroton	high blood pressure (diuretic/water pill)
Hytrin	high blood pressure (alpha blocker)
Hyzaar	high blood pressure (antihypertensive)
ibuprofen	inflammation; pain; fever (anti-inflammatory)
Imdur	heart problems; angina (coronary vasodilator)
Imitrex	migraine headaches (antimigraine)
Inderal	high blood pressure; heart problems; angina (beta blocker)
Indocin	osteoarthritis; pain (anti-inflammatory)
indomethacin	arthritis (anti-inflammatory)
Intal	asthma (mast cell stabilizer)
Iophen	cough (antitussive)
Isoptin	angina; high blood pressure; rapid heart rate
Isordil	heart problems; angina (coronary vasodilator)
isosorbide dinitrate	heart problems; angina (coronary vasodilator)
K-Dur	potassium replacement, taken with diuretics
K-Tab	potassium replacement, taken with diuretics

Keflex	infection (antibiotic)
Keppra	seizure disorder (anticonvulsant)
ketoconazole	fungal infection (antifungal)
ketorolac	pain management (anti-inflammatory)
Klonopin	seizure disorder (anticonvulsant)
labetalol	high blood pressure (beta blocker)
Lamictal	seizure disorder (anti-epileptic)
Lamisil	antifungal
Lanoxin	heart problems
Lasix	congestive heart failure (diuretic/water pill)
Lescol	high cholesterol (cholesterol lowering agent)
Levaquin	infection (antibiotic)
Levitra	erectile dysfunction
Levothroid	thyroid disease (thyroid hormone)
levothyroxine	thyroid problems (thyroid hormone)
Levoxyl	thyroid disease (thyroid hormone)
Lexapro	depression
Librax	peptic ulcer (anticholinergic)
Lipitor	high cholesterol (cholesterol lowering agent)
lisinopril	high blood pressure
lithium carbonate	behavioral disorders (antipsychotic)
Lodine	arthritis; pain (anti-inflammatory)
Loestrin Fe	birth control pills

Lomotil	diarrhea (antidiarrheal)
Lopid	high cholesterol (cholesterol lowering agent)
Lopressor	high blood pressure (beta blocker)
Lorabid	infection (antibiotic)
loracarbef	infection (antibiotic)
loratadine	allergies (antihistamine)
lorazepam	anxiety (sedative/antianxiety)
Lorcet	pain (narcotic analgesic)
Lortab	pain (narcotic analgesic)
Lotensin	high blood pressure (ACE inhibitor)
Lotrel	hypertension
Lotrimin	fungal infection (antifungal cream and ointment)
Lotrisone	fungal infection (antifungal cream)
lovastatin	high cholesterol (cholesterol lowering agent)
Lozol	congestive heart failure; high blood pressure
Lunesta	sleep aid
Luvox	Parkinson disease (anti-Parkinson)
Lyrica	nerve pain
Macrobid	urinary tract infection (antibiotic)
Macrodantin	urinary tract infection (antibiotic)
Maxzide	high blood pressure (diuretic/water pill)
meclizine	dizziness; vertigo; motion sickness (antiemetic)

medroxyprogesterone	gynecologic problems
meloxicam	inflammation; pain
metformin	diabetes
methadone	pain (narcotic analgesic); opiate withdrawal
methylphenidate	attention-deficit disorder; narcolepsy
methylprednisolone	anti-inflammatory
metoclopramide	gastric problems (antiemetic)
metoprolol tartrate	high blood pressure; heart problems (beta blocker)
metronidazole	infection (anti-infective)
Mevacor	high cholesterol (cholesterol lowering agent)
Micro-K	potassium replacement, taken with diuretics
Micronase	diabetes (oral antidiabetic)
milrinone	heart failure (vasodilator)
Minipress	high blood pressure (antihypertensive)
Minocin	infection (antibiotic)
minocycline	infection (antibiotic)
Miralax	constipation
Mirapex	Parkinson disease (anti-Parkinson)
Mircette	birth control pills
mirtazapine	anxiety; depression
Mobic	inflammation; pain
moexipril	high blood pressure
Monopril	high blood pressure
Motrin	inflammation; pain; fever

nabumetone	inflammation; pain (anti-inflammatory)
Namenda	Alzheimer disease
Naprosyn	inflammation; pain (anti-inflammatory)
naproxen	inflammation; pain (anti-inflammatory)
Nasacort	asthma; breathing problems (anti-inflammatory)
Nasonex	allergies (anti-inflammatory)
Necon	birth control pills
Neurontin	seizure disorders (anticonvulsant)
Nexium	gastric problems
Niaspan	high cholesterol
nifedipine	heart problems; angina (coronary vasodilator)
Nipride	heart failure (vasodilator)
Nitro-Dur	heart problems; angina (coronary vasodilator)
nitrofurantoin	urinary tract infection
nitroglycerin	heart problems; angina (coronary vasodilator)
nitroprusside	heart failure (vasodilator)
Nitrostat	heart problems; angina (coronary vasodilator)
nizatidine	ulcers (antiulcer)
Nizoral	fungal infection (antifungal)
Norco	pain (narcotic analgesic)
Normodyne	high blood pressure
nortriptyline	depression (antidepressant)

Norvasc	high blood pressure (calcium-channel blocker)
nystatin	fungal infection (antifungal)
omeprazole	ulcers, gastric problems (antiulcer)
Omnicef	infections (antibiotic)
Omnipen	infections (antibiotic)
ondansetron	nausea
Ortho-Cept	birth control pills
Ortho-Cyclen	birth control pills
Ortho-Novum	birth control pills
Ortho Tri-Cyclen	birth control pills
Oruvail	arthritis pain (anti-inflammatory)
oseltamivir	antiviral
oxaprozin	inflammation; pain; fever (anti-inflammatory)
oxcarbazepine	seizures
oxybutynin	bladder problems (antispasmodic)
oxycodone	pain (narcotic analgesic)
Oxy-Contin	pain (narcotic analgesic)
Pamelor	depression (antidepressant)
pantoprazole	gastric problems; ulcers
paroxetine	depression (antidepressant)
Pataday	allergies (antihistamine)
Patanol	allergies (antihistamine)
Paxil	depression (antidepressant)
Pediazole	infection (antibiotic)

penicillin	infection (antibiotic)
pentoxifylline	vascular disease (blood thinner)
Pepcid	ulcers; gastric problems (antiulcer)
Percocet	pain (narcotic analgesic)
Percodan	pain (narcotic analgesic)
Persantine	thromboembolism
phenazopyridine	urinary tract irritation, infection
Phenergan	nausea (antiemetic)
phenobarbital	seizure disorder (anticonvulsant)
phentermine	weight loss
phenytoin	seizure disorder (anticonvulsant)
Plavix	thromboembolism (antiplatelet)
Plendil	high blood pressure (calcium-channel blocker)
potassium chloride	potassium replacement, taken with diuretics
Prandin	diabetes (oral antidiabetic)
Pravachol	high cholesterol (cholesterol lowering agent)
prednisone	severe inflammation (anti-inflammatory)
Premarin	menopause; gynecological problems (estrogen)
Prempro	menopause; gynecologic problems
Prevacid	ulcers; gastric problems (antiulcer)
Prilosec	ulcers, gastric problems (antiulcer)
Primacor	heart failure (vasodilator)

Prinivil	high blood pressure (ACE inhibitor)
Pro-Banthine	peptic ulcer (anticholinergic)
Procan	rapid heart rate; tachycardia (antiarrhythmic)
Procardia	heart problems; angina (coronary vasodilator)
Proloprim	infection, mainly urinary tract (antibiotic)
promethazine	nausea (antiemetic)
Propacet	pain management (narcotic analgesic)
Propecia	hair loss
propofol	anesthetic
propoxyphene	pain management (narcotic analgesic)
propranolol	high blood pressure; heart problems; angina (beta blocker)
Proscar	prostate enlargement
Protonix	gastric problems
Proventil	breathing problems (bronchodilator)
Provera	gynecologic problems (progestogen)
Provigil	narcolepsy
Prozac	depression (antidepressant)
Pulmicort	asthma
Pyridium	urinary tract infections; pain
Quinaglute	ventricular arrhythmias (antiarrhythmic)
quinapril	high blood pressure (ACE)
ramipril	high blood pressure (ACE)
ranitidine	ulcers; gastric problems (antiulcer)
Relafen	inflammation; pain (anti-inflammatory)

Remeron	anxiety; depression (sedative)
Restoril	sleep disorders (hypnotic)
Retrovir	antiretroviral
Risperdal	psychological disorders (antipsychotic)
Ritalin	attention-deficit disorder; narcolepsy
Robaxin	muscle spasms (muscle relaxant)
Roxicet	pain management (narcotic analgesic)
Rythmol	heart problems; ventricular tachycardia
Sectral	high blood pressure (beta blocker)
Septra	infection (antibiotic)
Serevent	asthma; breathing problems (bronchodilators)
Seroquel	psychological disorders (antipsychotic)
sertraline	depression (antidepressant)
Serzone	depression (antidepressant)
simvastatin	high cholesterol
Sinemet	Parkinson disease (anti-Parkinson)
Sinequan	anxiety or depression (antidepressant)
Singulair	asthma
Skelaxin	muscle relaxant
Slo-Bid	breathing problems; asthma (bronchodilator)
Slow-K	potassium replacement, taken with diuretics
Soma	muscle spasms (muscle relaxant)
Spiriva	breathing problems

spironolactone	high blood pressure; heart failure (diuretic)
Suboxone	treatment of opioid dependence
sucralfate	ulcers (antiulcer)
Sular	high blood pressure
sulfamethoxazole	infection (antibiotic)
sulfasalazine	ulcerative colitis (antibacterial)
sulfisoxazole	infection (antibiotic)
Sumycin	infection (antibiotic)
Suprax	infection (antibiotic)
Sustiva	antiretroviral
Symbicort	asthma
Synthroid	thyroid disease (thyroid hormone)
Tagamet	ulcers; gastric problems (antiulcer)
Tamiflu	antiviral
tamoxifen	cancer (antineoplastic)
Tavist	allergies (antihistamine)
Tegretol	seizure disorder (anticonvulsant)
temazepam	insomnia (sedative)
Tenex	high blood pressure (alpha blocker)
Tenormin	high blood pressure; heart problems; angina (beta blocker)
Tequin	infection (anti-infective)
terazosin	high blood pressure (alpha blocker)
tetracycline	infection (antibiotic)
Theo-Dur	breathing problems (bronchodilator)

theophylline	breathing problems (bronchodilator)
Tiazac	high blood pressure
Ticlid	stroke (antiplatelet)
Tigan	nausea and vomiting (antiemetic)
Tofranil	depression (antidepressant)
Tolinase	diabetes (oral antidiabetic)
Topamax	seizures
Toprol	high blood pressure (beta blocker)
Toradol	short-term pain
tramadol	pain (analgesic)
trazodone	depression (antidepressant)
Trental	vascular disease (blood thinner)
triamterene	high blood pressure (diuretic)
Triavil	anxiety; depression (antidepressant)
Tricor	high triglycerides (antilipemic)
trimethoprim	infection, mainly urinary tract (antibiotic)
Trimox	infection (antibiotic)
Triphasil	birth control pill
Trivora-28	birth control pills
Tussionex	cough (antitussive)
Tylenol with codeine (Tylenol #3)	pain
Ultram	pain (analgesic)
valacyclovir	herpes (antiviral)
Valium	anxiety (antianxiety)

valproic acid	seizure disorder (anticonvulsant)
Valtrex	herpes (antiviral)
Vantin	infections (antibiotic)
Vasotec	high blood pressure; heart failure
Veetids	infection (antibiotic)
venlafaxine	depression (antidepressant)
Ventolin	breathing problems (bronchodilator)
verapamil	angina; high blood pressure; rapid heart rate
Viagra	erectile dysfunction
Vibramycin	infection (antibiotic)
Vicodin	pain (narcotic)
Vicoprofen	pain (narcotic analgesic)
Viramune	antiretroviral
Viread	antiretroviral
Voltaren	arthritis (anti-inflammatory)
Vytorin	high cholesterol
warfarin sodium	blood clots (blood thinner)
Wellbutrin	depression (antidepressant)
Xalatan	glaucoma
Xanax	anxiety; depression (sedative)
Xenical	weight loss
Xopenex	breathing problems
Yasmin	birth control
YAZ	birth control
Zantac	ulcers; gastric problems (antiulcer)

Zerit	antiretroviral
Zestoretic	high blood pressure
Zestril	high blood pressure (ACE inhibitor)
Zetia	high cholesterol
Ziac	high blood pressure (beta blocker, diuretic)
Zithromax	infection (antibiotic)
Zocor	high cholesterol (cholesterol lowering agent)
Zofran	nausea
Zoloft	depression (antidepressant)
zolpidem	sleep aid
Zomig	migraine headaches
zonisamide	seizures
Zovirax	herpes, shingles, chickenpox (antiviral)
Zyflo	asthma
Zyloprim	gout
Zyprexa	psychological disorders (antipsychotic)
Zyrtec	allergies (antihistamine)

Phone Numbers

Adult Protective Services _____

AIDS Information _____

Air Medical Service _____

Alzheimer's Information _____

American Red Cross _____

Animal Control _____

Battered Women's Hotline _____

Chemtrec: 1-800-424-9300 _____

Children's Services _____

CISM Team _____

Communications/Dispatch _____

Domestic Violence Center _____

Hazardous Materials Team _____

Health Department _____

Homeless Shelter _____

Infection Control Department _____

Medic Alert: 1-800-625-3780 _____

Medical Examiner/Coroner _____

Poison/Drug Information Center _____

Psychiatric Emergency Services _____

Rape/Sexual Abuse Crisis Center _____

SIDS Hotline _____

Suicide Prevention Hotline _____

Towing Service/Heavy Wrecker _____

Translators (note language) _____

Toxicologist _____

Hospital Phone Numbers and Radio Channels

Hospital Name	Medical Control Phone Number	Emergency Room Phone Number	Medical Control Radio Channel
	01 39		

Note: If the hospital has a dedicated phone number for contacting medical control, note this in the appropriate space. Otherwise, leave blank and use the regular emergency room phone number for communications. If the hospital has medical radio capability, note which radio channel to use.

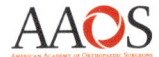

EMT Field Guide

THIRD EDITION

Fully updated to reflect the *National EMS Education Standards* and the 2015 CPR and ECC guidelines, this concise, indispensable resource provides easy access to the vital emergency information needed by BLS personnel. Color-coded tabs and a logical presentation of information enable BLS personnel to find the information they need when they need it most. An all-new section on the most common medical emergencies encountered in the field features relevant signs and symptoms and appropriate management steps and makes this a must-have resource for BLS providers.

The *Third Edition* features:

- Personalized forms
- Patient assessment tools
- Key medical and trauma emergencies
- CPR summary for adult and pediatric patients
- Pediatric guidelines
- General pharmacology for BLS providers
- Tips on ensuring safe transport

- HazMat identification tools
- Mass-casualty incident guidelines
- Tools to ensure proper and professional patient care reports
- Common prescription medications encountered in the field

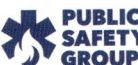

PUBLIC SAFETY GROUP

A DIVISION OF JONES & BARTLETT LEARNING

Market-leading EMS and Fire resources that go beyond initial training to support providers throughout every step of their education and careers.

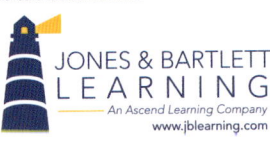

JONES & BARTLETT LEARNING

An Ascend Learning Company

www.jblearning.com

ISBN-13: 978-1-284-16091-8

9 781284 160918

90000